FACE READING
IN CHINESE MEDICINE

FACE READING
IN CHINESE MEDICINE

Lillian Bridges
The Lotus Institute
Kirkland, Washington

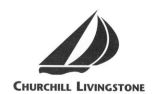

CHURCHILL LIVINGSTONE

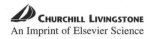

CHURCHILL LIVINGSTONE
An Imprint of Elsevier Science

11830 Westline Industrial Drive
St. Louis, Missouri 63146

FACE READING IN CHINESE MEDICINE   ISBN 0-443-07315-5

Distributed in the United Kingdom by Churchill Livingstone, Robert Stevenson House, 1-3 Baxter's Place, Leith Walk, Edinburgh EH1 3AF, Scotland, and by associated companies, branches, and representatives throughout the world.

Churchill Livingstone and the sailboat design are registered trademarks.

Library of Congress Cataloging in Publication Data

Bridges, Lillian.
   Face reading in Chinese medicine/Lillian Bridges.
      p. cm.
   Includes index.
   ISBN 0-443-07315-5 (pbk.)
      1. Physiognomy. 2. Facial exercises. 3. Facial expression. 4. Face—Care and hygiene. I. Title.
BF851.B69 2003
138–dc21   2003051494

Publishing Director: Linda Duncan
Publishing Manager: Inta Ozols
Associate Developmental Editor: Melissa Kuster Deutsch
Publishing Services Manager: Linda McKinley
Designer: Amy Buxton

Printed in the United States of America

Last digit is the print number: 9 8 7 6 5 4 3 2 1

Acknowledgments

This book took a very long time to write and a lot of wonderful clients and students passed through my life and influenced the way it all turned out. Thanks for all of your insightful questions. To all the Community Services Directors, Deans, and Conference Directors, thanks for hiring me. Special thanks go to Inta Ozals, my Publishing Manager, who could see what this book was supposed to be and took a chance on making it so. To Melissa Kuster, my Development Editor—your eye for detail and your witty emails always made editing a pleasure. To all of the staff at Elsevier who worked on this book, thanks for your input. To Kellie White, my Commissioning Editor, and to Kelly Mabie, my Production Editor from Graphic World, thanks for shepherding this book through the final stages of creation. I also have to applaud all the subjects in this book. Thanks for being so brave and beautiful too!

Personally, I have been blessed by having some extraordinary people as relatives. My greatest debt goes to my grandmother, Mary Lowe, my first and best teacher of face reading and ancient Chinese wisdom. I can never thank her enough. My father, Harold Rubright, had a dream of retiring so that he could write, but sadly never got the chance. He gave me the love of reading, learning, and writing and was my first teacher of psychology, medicine, and spirituality. I wish he were here to see how he inspired me. My beautiful and spirited mother, Lea, has always been an amazing catalyst for creativity and a champion for living your dreams. I could not have gone on with this project after some of those dark days if she hadn't said, "I know you can!" To my aunts and uncles, Pearl, Phillip, Ben, Alex, and Lily, thank you too. You never tired of my questions.

To all my close friends—you know who you are—thank you for believing in me. I owe particular thanks to Hannah Shearer, for her support and advice about the writing life and for being my companion on our early spiritual quests, and to Deborah Mayo, for always being there, reading every edit, giving great advice, and taking me shopping or out for tea whenever I needed a lift.

To my husband, Hal Bridges, thanks for the fabulous photos, putting up with my obsession, and your constant devotion. To Leslie Daff, thank you for your love and understanding; I'm so lucky that you are my sister. Thanks for my wonderful niece and nephew, Katie and Chuck Daff, too. My sons, Stephen and Alex Lesefko, are the reason I believe in miracles. They never held me back, always give me joy, and are the best gifts I have ever received. This book is for you.

Contents

Introduction

Facial diagnosis has a venerated and well-documented history in China that dates back thousands of years. It was originally used to diagnose illness as a part of Chinese Medicine and was one of the many techniques doctors used to avoid having to palpate the body. Perhaps you have seen the ivory statues of nude Chinese women reclining. These statues were used by female patients; they would point out where their pain was on the statue because it was considered unseemly for the doctor to touch the female patient. Instead, other techniques like pulse, tongue, smell, and facial diagnosis were used. Face reading became a common tool used in countless ways, from matchmaking to determining promotability in the government hierarchy.

Face reading is still used today by Chinese people everywhere but primarily as a fortune-telling tool because the face not only shows who someone is, but also shows what has happened to them. If they stay on the same track, it also shows where they are probably going. Therefore it can be used to predict the future with a fair degree of accuracy. Predicting what kind of illness a person is headed for is even easier because the indications can be found in facial features long before tests show what organs are compromised or diseased. Even now, it is possible to go to any Chinatown in North America and get your face read for a minimal cost; the face reader will tell you about your fate and destiny. In many ways, fortune tellers acted as good therapists and helped people with their emotional and physical problems. The only downside to face reading was the negative judgment and criticism that the "wrong" face or features could elicit.

Face reading is not limited to the Chinese alone, however. It has a long history in the Western world as well. The Greeks were known to have studied physiognomy; both Aristotle and Plato wrote about faces. Europe has had a long tradition of evaluating faces ever since. Phrenology—reading the bumps on one's head—was popular in both Europe and America in the eighteenth century, and one of America's most revered presidents, Abraham Lincoln, was known to have picked his cabinet members based on their faces. There is even an out-of-print Maytag Sales Manual from the early 1900s that shows how reading faces helps to sell appliances.

I learned face reading from my mother's Chinese family. It has been passed down for many generations and has always been used for medical diagnosis, fortune telling, or as a business tool. My grandmother was fortunate enough to have learned these ancient teachings from her father, who allowed her to learn about it because she was his favorite child. It was not common for girls to be taught this information in the apprenticeship method. Her father used face reading as a business tool. He was a very well-to-do banker in Shanghai and attributed his success in banking to his ability to read faces and personalities and to be able to decide whom to loan money to, for how long, and also how much to loan them!

My grandmother used face reading as a business tool, as well, helping her to successfully run a major sweater manufacturing business. She read everyone's face that came to her house and told them all about their personality, their abilities, their health, and their potential. I was fortunate to have had her as a constant presence in my life since the age of 5. I would go to her house every weekend and sit by her side and watch her read faces. Her home was like Grand Central Station, and everyone had to be read! It was a requirement for passing through, and when they came back she would reevaluate them.

My grandmother was a wise and wonderful woman, but she was also a savvy businesswoman (Color Plate 1). She found face reading to be an excellent tool for helping her deal with people. I chose to learn about face reading because I loved being around her. She fascinated me. She taught all of her six children to read faces; however, I am the only grandchild out of twenty who chose to learn it and use it and I have spent my entire career reapplying it to the field of Oriental Medicine.

Although I spent my childhood learning about faces, I didn't take it all that seriously until I realized that other people didn't read faces. For this, I owe a debt of thanks to my ex-husband. This poor man had to pass the test of my family before I was allowed to marry him, and this was no small feat! He is a very left-brained and logical engineer, but luckily had an open mind. When we started becoming serious about each other, I had to take him to my grandparent's house. We walked in the front door and my uncle shook his hand and then stared intently at his forehead and said, "Oh, you almost died when you were 24, what happened?" His mouth just dropped open and he asked, "How did you know that I almost died?" My uncle's reply was very simple, "Well, it's right there on your forehead."

At that point, I am sure that he thought he was marrying into a family of witches! The rest of my aunts and uncles proceeded to analyze him, evaluate him, and interrogate him. Ultimately, my grandmother gave me her approval with a few warnings about the differences in our personalities. By the time we left, he was in a state of shock. He wanted to know how they all knew so much about him. I tried to explain that this was just face reading and that I could do it, too. He encouraged me to start writing a book on the subject with lots of scientific validation; until that moment, I had never thought that face reading was an extraordinary ability. I believed that because my family did it, many other people must be able to read faces, too. I started my research over 20 years ago.

I researched ancient Chinese medical texts, interviewed a variety of family members and had them translate ancient texts, and pored over studies in medical and psychology journals. The more I looked, the more I found in Western science that backed up what the Chinese have always known.

I started teaching face reading soon after my initial period of research, starting out at metaphysical bookstores in the 1980s and proceeding to teach continuing education at community colleges and then at universities. I was invited to speak at my first medical conference in 1992, and since then have gone on to become a professor of Oriental Medicine both as a faculty member and as a visiting instructor. I speak at conferences around the world and have applied face reading in every way imaginable. I have taught businesspeople to use face reading in management, hiring, sales, and for international business communication. I have taught spa guests about beauty, health, and rejuvenation—otherwise known as "getting rid of wrinkles." I have even taught lawyers how to use face reading to pick juries and those in singles' groups how to pick a mate! I have taught doctors, nurses, and acupuncturists how to read illness from the face and developed a specialty of recognizing the psychological and emotional underlay of disease from the recognition of life patterns that appear on the facial map. Most important to me, though, is that I have passed on the ability to read faces to my two wonderful boys. It has been a fascinating journey and a totally unexpected career. If anyone had asked me 25 years ago what I would be doing with my life, I would never have answered "face reading"!

So what can you do with face reading? You have been reading faces since you were born. It is one of the first things that all human beings do. Babies are born with the ability to see about 18 inches away from the face, which, when held in the mother's arms, is the perfect position to read her expressions! Babies would rather look at faces than any other picture.[1]

We are wired to read faces, and we do so every day. We spend a great deal of time looking closely at someone's face to gauge even slight changes in expression that indicate an altered mood. We hear many references to the faces of others. We say things like "He has shifty eyes" or "She has such a stubborn chin." Our language is full of references to face reading: it is a primal and universal language. We have innate skills that let us read facial expressions. It is so deep-rooted that researchers have discovered that stroke victims who could not recognize their own faces in the mirror could still distinguish a smile from a frown. Face reading is a fundamental skill.

Other studies have shown that every major culture in the world uses the same basic expression to relay the same basic emotions. This is why communication can be accomplished in foreign countries even when people don't speak the language; they are reading expressions and faces! The face has so much to tell you that once you relearn and remember how to translate this universal language for your own use, you will be amazed at the amount of information each face contains.

The face is the most powerful communication tool we have. The face is the first thing we see and we spend the rest of our lives watching them. The face alone can communicate the impressive range of human emotions. This book can teach you the secrets of the ancient Chinese scholars and doctors. More specific than body

---

[1]Bower B: Faces of perception, *Sci News* 160(1), 2001.

language and much easier to apply than personality testing, reading faces can become an invaluable communication tool for your personal and business relationships. Most important, it is the window into the workings of the body and the mind. It is an ancient technique with many modern medical and psychological applications. My grandmother's legacy is now a gift of knowledge that I wish to share with you.

The Changing Face

"God has given you one face, and you make yourself another."
WILLIAM SHAKESPEARE, *HAMLET*, ACT III, SC. 1, LINE 150

You are your face. It is your identity. We carry pictures of ourselves on our driver's licenses, our passports, and now even on our credit cards. People recognize you faster from your face than from your name. Your face is scrutinized by others constantly. You express yourself through your face, and as you change, so does your face. The face is an external projection of your inner self and the reflection of your emotional world. The approximately 25 square inches of the face give more information about you than any other part of your body.

Your face is an intriguing combination of genetic structure, environmental influence, and markings caused by repetitive expression. It shows the world who you are, how you have felt, and what you are likely to feel again. It also shows what you have done and potentially where you can go. That's a lot to read in a very small area. How do you begin reading it?

My grandmother's favorite saying was "From birth until the age of 25, you have the face that your mother gave you. From 25 to 50, you create your own face. And, from 50 on, you have the face that you deserve!" She hastened to add that even after 50, you could change your face.

Most people believe that their face is primarily inherited, and heredity does play an important part in creating the structure of the face, as seen in Figure I-1. But what accounts for people starting to look more alike the longer they stay married, as seen in Figure I-2, or even stranger, people who start looking like their dogs?

Simply put, the longer you live with someone, the more emotions and expressions you share. These expressions change the markings on your face, and you end up living more often on the same emotional wavelength. You obviously have more control over what is on your face than you ever thought was possible. Over the

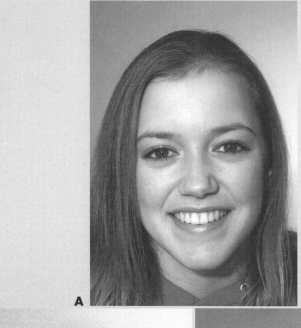

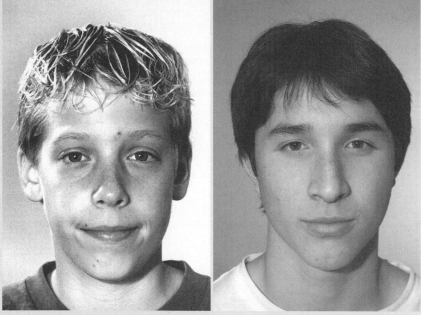

FIGURE I-1.   Faces Still Changing.   These three 15-year-olds are still carrying the faces their mothers gave them. Some of their features are already very distinctive, but their bone structure can be expected to develop further and will most likely increase the size of their chins and jaws. Also, the constant use of habitual expressions will not only mark their faces but also change the shape of their softer features such as their eyes and mouths.

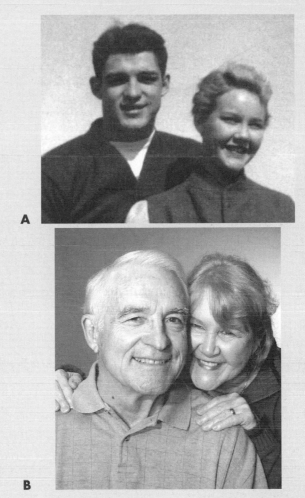

FIGURE I-2. Married Faces, Then and Now.   Faces lengthen as we grow older and become more lined, but this couple, soon to celebrate their 50th wedding anniversary, have even started looking more alike. This is after starting off together looking very different. Living together and sharing thoughts, experiences, and expressions have made their bond closer.

years, I have seen faces change so much that I have often been unable to recognize people I used to know well. I know my face has changed—hasn't yours?

At my 20-year high school reunion, I was more than a little shocked at how much my classmates had changed. If they hadn't been wearing name tags with their yearbook photos on them, I would have been stumped a number of times. Everybody looked so different. Then several women came over to me and, after telling me how great I looked, started asking me whether I had plastic surgery on my face. I was floored; I hadn't done a thing. Finally, one of them said, "I know what's different about you; you have so much more strength in your face now—you are so much more defined. You have bones now. What have you done to yourself?" I laughed as I finally understood and replied, "Oh, I earned those from suffering!"

As I looked down at my own yearbook picture, I realized how passive I had been at 18; my rounded chin, big eyes, and the overall softness were no longer evident. I had worn rose-colored glasses and was so sweet that I hardly dared to have an opinion in case I might offend someone who disagreed with me. Now, my friends can't believe that I was once so subservient. I currently have strong cheekbones, a very aquiline nose, an angled jaw, and much more of a chin. The world and my experiences have toughened me up. I grew these features the hard way, from life experiences that challenged me and helped me build my character. As I grow older, I look less and less like the passive young girl that I was, and I'm glad.

How do your features change? When I first started practicing face reading, I had no idea how much people could change their faces on purpose or even unconsciously. Over the years, I have seen eyebrows get thicker and finer, noses get fatter and skinnier, and cheekbones grow. I've come to the conclusion that the face is really like a hologram, a three-dimensional projection of our inner selves. It has led me to theorize that what is most important about the changing face is in the growth of the individual's spirit, essence, or soul. In fact, our genetics are a framework of existence, and our life experiences are a test of character with our soul's awakening as the reward. Let's start with the framework.

THE FACE YOU WERE BORN WITH

Every parent eagerly awaits the birth of a child. They can't wait to see whom the baby looks like. It's the great genetic lottery. Parents, grandparents, and other relatives all examine children to announce such things as "He looks just like his father at that age," or "She has her mother's eyes." They scrutinize and analyze. They pay close attention to the obvious signs of genetic relationship. One interesting study[1] recently noted that babies look more like their fathers at birth than they do at any other time in life so that the father will claim them and not reject them as someone else's child.

Looks are extremely important from the start. Parents are thrilled or alarmed at features that identify their babies as belonging to them. Think of some famous families known for some very unusual features, like the Hapsburgs and their notorious chin (or lack thereof). One of my former students worried and worried about her children inheriting her husband's protruding ears, and that turned out to be a dominant trait that both children got. She has already made plans to have them pinned back by the time they are 12. Some traits are very dominant and are major clues to personality traits, expressed or unexpressed. I'm always meeting people who deny that they have the bad temper that I have recognized from very heavy eyebrows. After a little coaxing, they will admit that they control their anger

---

[1]Christenfeld NJ, Hill EA: Whose baby are you? *Nature* 378:669, 1995.

most of the time, but when they blow, watch out! We deny a lot of traits and tend to use those few familiar and comfortable ones of which people approve.

Each person's inheritance is a complex mixture of his or her ancestors' traits. Geneticists have theorized that we carry up to 14 generations of traits. That means we inherit a lot of things from a lot of people whom we don't even know. Parents, however, are always saying things such as "You are just like your father!" No, you're not, you can't be. You are you, and it takes a lot of work to bring out and balance all the traits that you are carrying around. You may have your father's stubborn chin, and you can be stubborn like your father, but what happens when you also have your mother's quick temper, your grandmother's kind eyes, and your grandfather's sense of justice?

This mixed bag of traits explains why siblings in one family can look so different. My two sons look and act so differently that people think they have different fathers. Their combination of traits makes my older son look tall, dark, and exotic and my younger son look like the traditional image of the all-American boy, with fair skin and freckles on his nose.

I think we spend most of our lives figuring out who we are and then deciding what to do about it. The inherited traits are very valuable because they provide predispositions for behavior. We can carry traits that we may or may not use. I like my youngest son's attitude. In the second grade, he had to write a report about ancestors. He said, "My hair looks like my grandma's, my forehead and my ears look like my Dad's. My eyes and nose look like my Mom's, but my smile is all mine!" It was refreshing to know that he feels that he belongs to all of his relatives and yet knows that he has expressions that are unique to him.

Even identical twins have their differences (Figure I-3). Although they share the same DNA, they cannot possibly have exactly the same environment, which accounts for variations in their personalities and therefore their expressions.[2] One of the oldest tenets of genetics was that you could not pass on acquired traits. This has now been determined to be a false statement. Your DNA changes as you do. For example, recent studies[3] have shown that mutations can occur in DNA from exposure to radiation, and these mutations can be passed on to future generations. We are obviously not just our inheritance. We are so much more. What else is there that makes you who you are?

THE FACE YOU CREATE

Remember that saying your mom was so fond of, "Don't make that face, it will freeze that way?" Well, guess what? She was right. If you make any expression over and over again, for years, it will mark your face. Most of us are creatures of habit, and we tend to use our favorite expressions repeatedly. Frankly, I think the face

---

[2]Glass J: Nature vs. nurture, *Parenting Magazine*, www.parenting.com, 1999.
[3]Kirby A: Chernobyl children show DNA changes, *BBC News Online*,
http://news.bbc.co.uk/1/hi/sci/tech/1319386.stm, 2001.

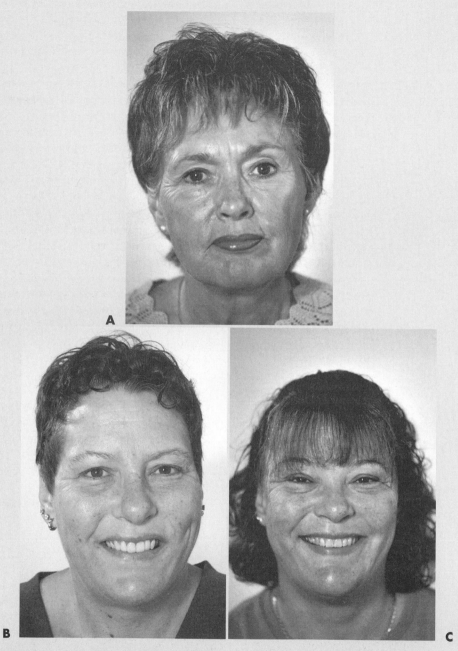

FIGURE I-3.   Related Faces.   This mother and her twin daughters share traits in common; for example, their eyebrows, cheekbones, and chins are similar. But as you can see, even identical twins have ended up looking different as a result of individual and varied life experiences.

just gets tired of working so hard and decides to take a shortcut and leave the expression there. And studies of brow lifters, squinters, and frowners have proven that expressions cause lines on the face. So, if you don't like the way your face is getting marked, stop making those expressions!

Human beings are capable of a great range of expressions. Anthropologists have studied every major culture in the world and discovered that we all use the same basic expressions for the same basic emotions. We are all wired the same under the skin. That's why we can understand the expressions of other people in the world. It is a universal language.

I have a slightly different perspective about wrinkles. I like them. I think they are fascinating and show how you have felt in the past and what you have lived through. They give me many clues to how often you smile, how intense or impatient you can be, how sad your life has been, and so on. I think lines can be very attractive and show that you've lived life. Vanity prevents me from saying that I like all the wrinkles I have on my face. Getting them is inevitable, but you do have control over how many you have and where they are. What makes some people get so many wrinkles and others so few?

People who don't wrinkle very much have several things in common. First is the quality of their skin. Thicker, oilier skin just doesn't wrinkle as easily. It holds those lines at bay for a longer time. They will eventually get the same wrinkles as everyone else when their skin gets drier and thins out more. Thinner, fragile skin lines very easily and must be protected. Remember when people used to rave about beautiful English skin? It is beautiful skin and was even more so before the advent of forced-air heating that started drying out the environments. The damp climate and gray skies of England protected those lovely delicate complexions. Sun damage takes a heavy toll on the face. A common misconception is that the sun causes wrinkles. The sun does not cause wrinkles to form. The sun causes wrinkles that are already present or developing from expressions to become more pronounced and deeper. It is like tanning leather. Your skin ages prematurely, dries out, and loses elasticity and the grooves get carved in. My son used to call wrinkles "scratches" on the face.

There are many current fads that supposedly remove and minimize wrinkles, from expensive skin creams to electrical impulses zapping your facial muscles to injection of a variety of strange substances. Expensive skin creams don't work much better than inexpensive ones. Despite all the micronutrients and additives that are supposed to be absorbed by the skin, moisturizers are designed to keep the moisture in your skin that you already have. Being hydrated on the inside is more important. Creams don't really add much from the outside; they are just another protective barrier.

Some people are strong proponents of facial exercises that are supposed to eliminate wrinkles. However, they cause overuse of facial muscles and skin that ultimately will make the face more lined down the road. The ancient Chinese always believed that expressions needed to come from the rising of *qi*, or energy caused by an emotion. When you fake an expression, you are wasting energy. Facial exercises will temporarily make your face look better because they increase blood supply to the face. However, they eventually will cause the very problems that they are trying to fix. In addition, the physiology of facial muscles is very different from that of other muscles in the body in the way they are attached. Using them does not strengthen them; it weakens them and causes more lines.

As for injections of substances such as collagen and BoTox, my advice is to be very careful. Allergies occur with collagen. BoTox is inactive Botulism toxin; were it active, it would kill the person injected. Although it is inactive, it could still compromise the user's immune system, and the side effects are not completely known. Besides that, every client I have seen who had this done had a frozen look to their skin and paralysis of the facial muscles in the treated area. I've even heard of women who were unable to close their eyelids! It is injected most often between the eyebrows, a minor liver area, resulting in a look of frozen skin. Does this lead to a frozen liver too? It is wiser to learn how to lessen wrinkles in a more natural way.

I have even heard of people implanting GoreTex in their lips to make them look fuller and more kissable. In reality, implanting GoreTex in the lips makes it hard or even painful to kiss, and frankly, this is thus false advertising. Full lips are a sign of sensuality, but if people want to look more sensual, they should cultivate their sensuality. The best way I know to plump up the lips is to kiss more! Kissing is a prescription in my practice.

Most of the lines that are caused by expressions are vertical. They are also fairly easy to remove or lessen in severity. My mom has a great technique. She uses ordinary tape. She puts pieces of tape over a wrinkle she doesn't like and leaves it there. Every time the tape pulls, she stops and asks herself, "What am I feeling right now? Why am I feeling this? Do I need to feel this, or can I let it go?" She then achieves insight into her reactions and unlearns some bad emotional habits. Frankly, many wrinkles are just patterns of behavior that have become ingrained and end up marking the face. She has lessened many wrinkles by this technique, although I advise that you do this in the privacy of your own home!

As for other ways not to get wrinkles, there are several types of people who don't wrinkle very much. The first type is the person who doesn't feel very much and therefore doesn't express very much. Think of a man who is always "in his head" or a woman who is "out of her body." These people are not emotionally present; therefore, they don't mark very much. They stay unwrinkled a lot longer than most people, but there is danger in living this way because they don't learn the skills to deal with life. They are usually unprepared for emotional traumas and have trouble coping. It is often amazing how much they suffer when they encounter such a trauma and how much they mark their faces. They seem to age overnight. This is the advantage in suffering when you are young. It may cause lines early, but it keeps you from getting lines later. You get to learn how to deal with life while you are still resilient.

The second type of person who doesn't wrinkle much is the one who is reclusive and lives away from the stresses of the world. Monks are a good example. They tend to have serene faces with few lines. Because their major needs are taken care of, their lives are sheltered. They have also chosen a spiritual life that involves a lot of contemplation and are less affected by the dramas of the world. They look otherworldly because they are. Stress definitely accelerates the aging process, and it is almost impossible to live in the modern world without a great deal of stress. Studies have shown that individuals who live in the country have fewer wrinkles than those who live in the city. Urban living is exciting, although it takes a toll on the body, and most people who live there are stimulated and energized from it. A balanced life might include frequent retreats to the country to destress and dewrinkle.

The third type of person who tends to have few wrinkles is one who does not hold onto past traumas. Many people cling to the wounds of the past and torment themselves continuously. My grandmother used to say that it didn't really matter what happened to you in life; it mattered how you felt about it and how you dealt with it. She was good at rising above things and looking at them from a higher perspective. She was a big believer in letting go of past hurts. One of the more recent expressions she would have loved was, "There is no such thing as a bad emotion—the only bad emotions are stuck emotions." Stuck emotions can cause many health problems and lines on the face. My grandmother had her share of tragedies and disasters. She once commented that, from the time she was born in China until the time she left, there was always a war going on. She had a child die in her arms in front of a hospital that wouldn't admit her daughter because my grandmother had forgotten to bring her purse. And yet she was capable of forgiving and releasing old hurts. She held no grudges and wanted no revenge. She died in her eighties with amazingly few lines and a very serene face, proof to me that letting go lessens lines.

What happens when people deliberately change their face with plastic surgery? This is a question that I have been asked repeatedly. I am not opposed to plastic surgery. It is a useful tool, especially when used for reconstruction and repair. As for minimizing noses, adding chins, and facelifts, I have mixed feelings. If people really wants to change their face this way, that's great; it's their body. However, I always recommend that people know what they are doing before they do it. There are consequences to changing the face in such a drastic manner.

Let's start with a face lift. Studies show that 5 to 7 years after someone has a face lift to remove wrinkles, it has to be done again. People get lines in the same places they had them before because they haven't changed their expressions. The face lift causes the skin to lose its natural elasticity, which could have been regained with a little work. However, if someone has reached the point of no return, if the wrinkles are very deep and there are very many, this may be the only recourse that gives the person back a sense of youth or beauty. Be aware that the younger an individual is at the time of the face lift, the more likely it will need to be repeated. Also, face lifts often create an unnatural looking mask that takes away much of the character of the face.

As for nose jobs, these are much more invasive, often involving cutting into bone and changing the whole balance of the face. They are also most often done in adolescence, when the nose is the largest feature on the face. The large nose is often blamed as the reason someone doesn't have enough confidence, isn't attractive enough, or isn't popular. Teenagers want to fit in and don't enjoy looking different. Large noses give the appearance of power. When the powerful nose is bobbed or shortened, the ability to act powerfully becomes diminished.

I know many women in their forties who had nose jobs as girls and have grown into women who would be very powerful but aren't allowed to be because they look too "cute" and aren't taken as seriously. Many of them eventually miss their large noses. Some people who have nose jobs are trying to take away the ethnicity of their nose. However, noses are the bridge on your face between other easily identifiable features. Ethnicity is something people become proud of as they get older.

Eye lifts are probably my favorite form of cosmetic surgery. Drooping eyelids can impede the vision. The very delicate skin has been overused because the individual tries to keep others out by narrowing the eyes. This occurs when someone has been heavily criticized or has tried to be overly analytical. "Tucking" the eyelid removes the mistrustful look and makes a person look more open and receptive. I have seen good results from this surgery, but I recommend doing the upper eyelids only. Removing bags has resulted in many cases of adrenal deficiency because of the use of lasers in an area of the face involving the kidneys and adrenal glands.

Homogenizing beauty is a danger in our society, and the cult of beauty has undermined many people's confidence in their personal and unique attractiveness. My wish is that plastic surgeons would make their patients aware of some of the ramifications of the changes they induce. Congruity of the personality and the structure of the face make us trust those whose face is consistent with their expressions. People who don't look the way they act can be misunderstood. My grandmother's name for people who have plastic surgery was "soft ears." These are people who care too much what others think and become what other people or society wants them to be. They listen to other people's opinions instead of trusting in themselves.

Luckily, most people are happy with the changes they make to their face when they have plastic surgery, and that's great. If you must have surgery, look for surgeons who are artists and perfectionists, who can sculpt features that blend and modify slightly rather than change the original intent.

If you can, learn to love the features that you have. Societal ideas of beauty come and go. What's in now will be out later. All features have special meaning and, when looked at as a whole, have a kind of symmetry and beauty that needs to be honored, appreciated, and understood. I'll never forget the day I met one of the ugliest men I have ever seen. Every feature on his face was unattractive, and yet his face was comfortable to look upon because everything matched. Because his face was so congruent, he was considered not only attractive, but lucky too! Since then, I have tried to teach my students to love their faces and themselves. I ask them to tell me whether they have any feature on their face that they hate, and I tell them what is wonderful about it.

1 / *The Facial Map*

"A man finds room in the few square inches of his face for the traits of all his ancestors; for the expression of all his history and his wants."
RALPH WALDO EMERSON, *BEHAVIOR*, "THE CONDUCT OF LIFE"

The face is a topographic map of personality, past experiences, and future potential. Most important, the face shows what is going on inside the body and in the mind, all of which change the landmarks. When I first learned about face reading, my grandmother talked about features being "mountains" and "rivers." The mountains are the hard features that are composed of bone—the forehead, the cheekbones, the nose, the chin, and the jaw. These features create the structure and foundation of the face and have personality traits associated with them such as stubbornness, willpower, bossiness, and ambition. The mountains are tied to the development of fundamental *yang qi* (the cosmic father), and the rivers to fundamental *yin qi* (the cosmic mother) *in utero*. Very strong *yang* traits show strength of character. Therefore people with large mountains would be very set in their ways and live out in the world.

Rivers are the soft features and exude fluid (the ears, eyebrows and eyes, nostrils and groove, and mouth). These features represent feelings. Large *yin* features indicate strength of emotions including traits such as generosity, sensuality, and sadness. People with large rivers are very emotional, expressive, and creative. They live a more internal life and are more malleable and changeable, depending on their moods.

The following describes a typical but partial reading by my grandmother. A man from Florida walked into her house; he was a potential new salesman for a company. He had a huge nose coming off his rather flat, narrow face and small eyes and mouth. My grandmother clucked when she saw him and said, "Oh my, what a solitary mountain." I asked her what she meant, and she replied, "Well, he has such a large mountain of a nose, which gives him a very large ego. He wants to succeed and have power at all costs. But he has no friends. There are no other mountains to keep him company [which meant that he had weak cheekbones and no chin or jaw to speak of and therefore had questionable ethics and no shame]. He doesn't even have any water to water the trees, so he is a bald mountain [which meant that he wasn't emotional or generous enough to have friends]. He will be a successful salesman, but he will always be a lonely man."

Another reading about rivers from my grandmother: A very pretty woman came in with a powerful-looking man. She had known my mother from school in China, but they hadn't seen each other since they were children. My grandmother clucked again. She said, "Oh dear, what a muddy river." I asked her what she meant. She first made me look at her hands. "Those are the hands of a mistress. She would rather be a mistress than work hard for a living." In fact, the man who brought her was married to someone else.

Then, my grandmother pointed out her very small nose in a broad face. She said that a nose that small was a sign of a person who would always be supported by someone else. She kindly pointed out that I did not have that kind of nose! Then, she made me aware of her very large eyes, large nostrils, and a cupid's-bow mouth. The eyes showed how emotional this woman was, the nostrils showed how much money she spent, and the mouth was an example of a petulant, self-indulgent woman. My grandmother said, "She is so emotional that her rivers wash all the dirt from the small mountains [meaning she didn't have a very strong character]. She is a muddy river because she lives by her feelings, always changes her mind, and uses manipulation instead of power to get her way." I was amazed at the assessment and, over time, have realized how accurate the reading of mountains and rivers alone can be.

Reading mountains and rivers requires taking an inventory of what features are the strongest on a face and looking at the balance between the two. For example, I have a relatively small face with a strong forehead (it is rounded), a strong nose, prominent cheekbones, and a moderately strong chin and jaw. I probably have more character than I need. Luckily, I also have large eyes and a large mouth, so I have some emotionality to back those up. I am weighted more heavily toward being mountainous and stand firm most of the time in my beliefs, ethics, and principles. My uncle informed me when I was 16 that I would always work for a living to support myself, even if I got married, so I had better get ready—he was right. The downside of having strong mountains means that you have to work very hard or you have struggled through some very hard character-building experiences. The good news is that mountainous people like to work hard and usually succeed because of their drive.

Larger, softer river features on a larger face indicate a life of more ease and less struggle. These people tend to be helped by others. Things come more easily, and emotions are more transitory, so suffering does not persist as long or penetrate as deeply. Curiously, every woman or man I know with this kind of face shape has been supported either by a spouse or by wealthy parents. One woman I know with this face shape was being supported by her two ex-husbands and had a live-in boyfriend who cooked, cleaned, and gave her massages! I asked her the secret to her pampered lifestyle, and she said, "I'm just lucky, I guess." The downside for river people is that they end up becoming dependent. The good news is that they get to live a more comfortable, pleasurable life.

Mountains and rivers are the topographic map of the face. Even more specific is the reading of age positions, which is like reading a map that gives you the placement of cities along a highway. Specific incidents mark specific places, recording the important events of a person's life.

THE AGE POSITIONS

The ancient Chinese believed that the face records the life experiences of an individual and the effects of these experiences on the psyche and the body, similar to tracing on a road map a route taken in the past. The facial map was originally composed of 150 age positions. The specific places on the facial map marked ages from conception to 150 years old, what the ancients believed was the possible life span of a human being. The oldest person known died recently at 122 years old. Scientists are now validating that this increased life span is possible but difficult to achieve: The average person in the United States lives to be only 78 years old. I use the map with 100 years on it because it is much more realistic to strive to become a centenarian (Figures 1-1 and 1-2).

Each child is born with a potential to live a given life span, and each child's battery (the kidney *jing*) is fully charged. Over time, overuse and depletion of this fundamental inherited *qi*, or life force energy, causes aging and disease. One of the most important tenets in Chinese medicine is to conserve this *jing*. Whenever something traumatic or stressful occurs in a person's life, the face marks a specific place because the *jing* has been affected. The life experience markings are primarily horizontal. Over time, the face shows most of the major traumas that have occurred and at the age when they happened. Knowing how to read these markings can help you track the patterns in a person's life. Western science has come up with an explanation of why we remember all these traumas; the Chinese show how to read them from the face.

As a defense mechanism, the instinctive part of the brain, the amygdala, has the ability to store emotional memories, which help by warning us so we can prevent a similar trauma from happening again. Because of the desire to avoid the recurrence of past events, people shut themselves off from learning the lesson of the experience and end up living reactively. Ironically, by trying to avoid repeating the experience, people actually attract and re-create similar experiences. People end up living in patterns that keep coming back to haunt them. It usually takes many repetitions before someone even recognizes the pattern and much willpower to avoid falling into the same trap again and again.

Much study has been done on the amygdala and its role as an early warning device for perceived potential pain and trauma. The amygdala is an almond-shaped structure on top of the brainstem at the bottom of the limbic system. This part of the brain is tied directly to the nose and eyes through the thalamus and is responsible for the ability to feel fear, rage, competition, or cooperation and to cry tears. Joseph LeDoux of the Center for Neural Science at New York University is the pioneer in this field of study. He has found that the amygdala can take over control of the body and its reactions before the neocortex has a chance to

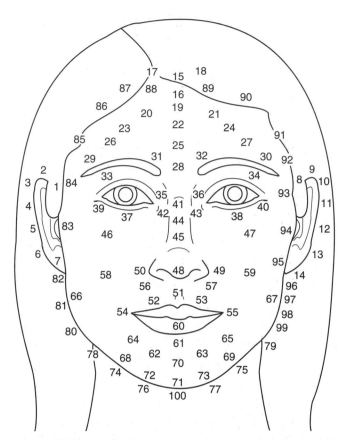

FIGURE 1-1.   The Facial Map—Female.   Numbers indicate Chinese age. Subtract 1 year for Western age.

respond.[1] The amygdala relays emergency information. It is responsible for emotional reactions without any conscious information or understanding. This demonstrates that the emotions have a way of being activated independently and that vivid emotional memories are stored in the amygdala.

When I was 8 years old, I got a very bad case of the stomach flu. My mother always fed me homemade chicken soup when I was sick, but this time she was in a play and made me instant chicken noodle soup, which I proceeded to throw up for days. To this day, I cannot stand the smell of instant chicken broth; it makes me nauseated. This is my amygdala at work. It has identified the smell of instant chicken soup as a potential poison and is warning me to stay away so that I will be safe. I know in my neocortex that there is nothing wrong with instant chicken soup, but my amygdala is somehow not getting retrained. The amygdala remembers all associated clues that accompany a traumatic or stressful event, which is why you may love the smell of your lover's cologne until he breaks up with you, at which point you can't stand

---

[1]LeDoux JE: Emotion and the limbic system concept, *Concepts in Neuroscience* 2:169-199, 1991.

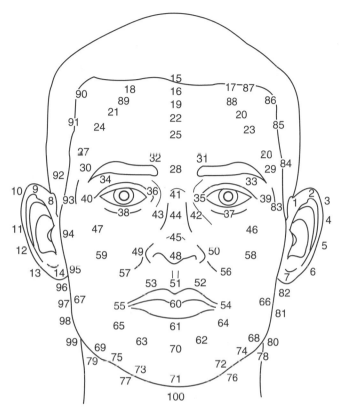

FIGURE 1-2.   The Facial Map—Male.   Numbers indicate Chinese age. Subtract 1 year for Western age.

it. It has become associated with the pain of the breakup. We have all experienced things like this.

Resisting your patterns encourages them to happen again. For example, I have had many female clients who have sworn that they will never marry domineering and controlling men. What do they do? They marry domineering and controlling men just like their fathers; they marry men the who are the exact opposite—the man who dominates through his passivity by forcing her to act like the dominator; or they marry men who get sick, and their lives become dominated by the circumstances of the illness. One way or another, they keep on repeating their pattern until they realize from where it stems. When they are able to recognize the issue when it returns, they can choose to deliberately step out of the pattern. Tests will come their way, because it takes a lot of work to overcome issues. The facial map helps show you where the issues begin and when they recur.

Any traumatic or stressful event is remembered by the amygdala, and the pain of that event can be a physical or psychological memory; the amygdala does not distinguish between the two. Memories that are preverbal—before the age of 3—are more firmly implanted in this part of the brain, and that is one of the reasons our most primal or core issues are so hard to work with, things like phobias and our relationship with food and love.

The problem with the amygdala is that by storing important emotional memories, it helps set up a belief system that results in a life lived reactively instead of with conscious intent. Because we try so hard to avoid recurrence of past hurts, we actually magnetize them back to us by our fear. That fear sets us up to create similar emotional experiences by our avoidance. Ultimately, the pattern that is set blocks *qi* and leads to specific diseases. At some point, we all need to overcome our issues and live a life we choose rather than one to which we react.

The facial map has an amazing ability to show people when in their life traumatic or stressful incidents occurred (at what approximate age), how severe they were, and when the pattern repeats. Interestingly, good and bad stress make the same kinds of marks. The ancient Chinese cautioned that getting too excited is bad for your health. It doesn't matter what happens to you; it only matters how you feel about it; it is the perception of the event that marks the face. There should be no judgment or comparisons made. Everyone has different levels of sensitivity and abilities to cope. I have seen similar depth of markings in someone whose best friend moved away in third grade and in another person who was involved in a bad accident at the same age.

The ancient Chinese started looking for markings from the time of conception. They believed that the *in utero* experience is one of the most important times in a person's life and considered it the first year. The events, conditions, and traumas of this period and the birth experience itself are the foundation for the expression of genetic structure and constitution. The markings on the ear reflect the mother's emotional state during pregnancy.

My grandmother used to say that the personality of a baby was affected by the personality of its mother while she was pregnant. This is one of those old wives' tales that has recently been proved true by modern scientists. Neuropeptides (the emotional messengers of the brain) are transmitted via the bloodstream across the placental barrier and end up in the baby's bloodstream, thus affecting the child's future moods. Furthermore, when a woman experiences significant stress while pregnant (events such as a parent or spouse dying, being in an accident, or getting very sick), the blood flow to the fetus constricts. At this time, because blood is food and food equals love and nurturing, the fetus goes into distress and ends up being born very tough. These babies have strong survival skills (high Apgar scores) but are nonbonders. They have poor ability to connect emotionally or physically. They often dislike touching and become difficult and angry children.

Many issues start *in utero*. Feelings of all kinds are transmitted and end up lodging in the baby's body, waiting to be recalled and turned into faulty beliefs. For those who are skeptical about this, scientists have discovered that so much is transferred to the fetus *in utero* that specific flavors from food the mother ingests get passed on and end up in the amniotic fluid to be tasted by the fetus. This accounts for a great number of food preferences, sensitivities, and cravings that cannot be fought.

The *in utero* experience starts marking on the ear—the right ear for women and left ear for men (this involves the *yin* and *yang* of the face), as shown in Figure 1-3.

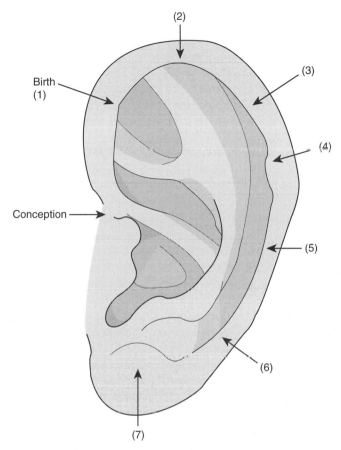

FIGURE 1-3.   Ear Map.   Numbers indicate Chinese age. Subtract 1 year for Western age. Start counting on right ear for women and left ear for men.

First look for the place where the upper and lower parts of the ear attach to the face. Right above this area is the place where conception is shown, and the first half-inch above that is the gestation period culminating in birth. Any marking, indentation, notch, groove, thinned-out area, wrinkle, spot, or discoloration has a meaning. For example, many people who were unwanted have a thinning of this area, whereas wanted babies or easy pregnancies (a good *in utero* experience) are wide and unmarked. Also, difficult births mark. I have seen veining on the ear as an indication of lack of oxygen, and a hole (literally) or an indentation indicating a physically traumatic birth (e.g., being stuck in the birth canal for a long time, which usually leads to claustrophobia).

In general, each time period is approximately ½ inch apart around the ear from conception to age 7 (Chinese age, age 6 in Western terms) on one ear, and 8 to 14 on the other ear (Chinese ages, age 7 to 13 in Western terms). Bumps or protrusions are considered positive and beneficial periods. Bumpiness indicates a period that is rocky, both good and bad. Basically, what goes up must go down, and that includes moods. Holes or notches indicate a very specific incident that caused trauma, usually physical. This could be an accident, an injury, physical abuse, an operation, etc.

Ears that look as though the cartilage gets thinner or is cut away show that this period was difficult because something important was taken away. For example, it may represent the death of a parent or grandparent or loss of attention because of a sibling's birth. When the ear looks as if it has been pushed down or pinched, it means that this was a suppressive period. This may been a time of much discipline or could indicate circumstances such as war or poverty that press down on the human spirit. Any marking on the ear needs to be evaluated.

One of my early issues involves my relationship with food, and I had no conscious memory about the original event that started my pattern. I have always had a great love of food, both cooking it and eating it. I love to shop for food, and I think about it all the time. I just assumed it was a pleasant hobby until I became a single mother. At that time money was very tight, and I panicked frequently about how to pay all the bills. But, whenever I had any money, the first thing I would do was go grocery shopping and buy way too much food. I didn't need it all, but I felt that I had to have it to feel safe. I sometimes would buy groceries first instead of paying the phone bill. I had an irrational terror of starving to death. I had never had a lack of food that I knew of, and food had always been a pleasure, not an issue—at least that was what I thought.

I called my mother and asked her if I had ever had a problem with eating, or if I had gone hungry at some time in my past, and her comment was, "Oh, didn't I ever tell you...." I love when she says that because inevitably it was something she never told me and something that I really wanted to know! Apparently, when I was born, my father was working for the CIA in Washington, D.C. My parents were living in Virginia at the time, and my mother, who is Chinese, was very far away from any of her family members in Los Angeles who might have given her advice or help. She was totally unprepared for the demands of a new baby, and she asked the doctor how often to feed me. He was a strong proponent of schedules, and he told her 10 minutes every 4 hours. He meant 10 minutes on each breast, but she took it as 10 minutes total and fed me 5 minutes on each side. I started screaming and crying because I was hungry, and she was beside herself. She didn't know what to do or what was wrong. She decided to hire a nanny and ended up getting a wonderfully warm woman who took one look at me and said, "This child is starving, we've got to feed her more." She started me on formula and I became a happy and contented baby. Six months after that, my family moved to Japan and I promptly began to feed myself Japanese food.

Well that got me to start thinking. I did have the markings on my right ear during the first year of my life indicating something was taken away; I had no idea it was food! And this food issue had come up repeatedly in my life. I always carried food around with me in case I got hungry. I was known for keeping snacks in my dorm room at college, and I would panic if I skipped a meal. I also got very cranky if I didn't eat. The aftereffects of my very brief period of food deprivation had made me live according to my pattern. I had just hired a nanny to watch my kids, and my first thought when I hired her was that she would feed my kids! According to my mother, she looked just like the one I had in Virginia that I didn't even remember having.

After having worked on my food issue for many years, I can honestly say that I am much calmer about food. I still crave Japanese food when times get stressful. It somehow just makes me feel safe and nurtured. My food issues have gotten better—they certainly don't run my life anymore. But food is still an important part of my life, and I'm always prepared to feed myself and everybody else. If there is ever a major disaster, come over to my house. I could feed a lot of people for at least a month with my fully stocked cupboards. But I now pay the phone bill first before I go grocery shopping. At this point, food brings pleasure instead of panic!

We all have many issues from the past, and they are worth finding out about. Interview your parents, siblings, and other relatives, and you will discover many of the reasons why you do what you can't help doing.

There are many issues to which we are predisposed because of the circumstances of our lives. Over the years, I have noticed that premature babies grow up to have major issues with time. They are usually very early or very late because they live according to a different clock. They tend to be late bloomers. Babies who aren't picked up or held have issues with affection. Babies who were left to cry believe that their needs won't get met when they speak. Many issues that affect our lives every day stem from events of which we have no memory because they occurred when we were so young.

Many previous issues repeat on a regular basis or cycle, which causes the ears to mark in a very similar way and in the same place on the other. Symmetric markings may suggest that they reflect the genetic structure of the ear, but it may just be a repeated pattern or the potential for a repeat of the pattern. Two bumps at 3 and 10 will look the same because something beneficial that occurred at 3 can often have a repeat performance 7 years later. Many of these markings that are made before you reach that age were set up *in utero* as an issue with a specific "shelf life."

Much like a milk carton that gives you an expiration date, the body is willing to hold onto certain emotions for only a set time, depending on the strength of the organ that is holding the emotion for you. When it is time for that issue to reemerge, almost anything can trigger it. Like the straw that breaks the camel's back, we often find issues reappearing even though the circumstances are not that similar to those that sparked the original occurrence because the associated feelings are similar. Ultimately, if you don't process these issues and free yourself from their hold, it takes a toll on your body. The longer someone waits to deal with an issue, the more likely it is to affect the person's energy. It is better to discover your issues earlier rather than later, because you have more energy to deal with them when you are younger.

One of my students gave me proof that the ears mark with childhood trauma. She was a pretty young woman about the age of 19 who had come to a Golden Path workshop. In that course, I require students to bring baby pictures of themselves to help them start tracking their life issues. She brought in pictures of when she was born and it was very clear that she had smooth unmarked ears. She had gone through a very traumatic period from the age of 3 until she was about 8 with chronic ear infections to the point that she had to have surgery and lost part of her hearing ability. As could be seen on her ear in person and in later photographs, she had marked the ear with repeated notches that were not there earlier. Trauma had changed the shape of her ears.

Let me give you another example of how issues keep coming back and continue to mark the face as the lessons are learned. I once had a client named John who came to see me because he knew I helped people recognize their issues. He was suffering from severe back spasms and had heart problems. John told me that everyone was always leaving him: his two wives, his kids, and his business partner. Now that he was engaged to a woman he really wanted to stay with, he was terrified that she might leave him too. John wanted help discovering the source of his problems, and he wanted to learn how to work through them.

In tracking John's patterns, I discovered that his father had died when he was 5 years old. This marked very heavily on the side of his left ear. There was a carved out section that showed something had been taken away. But the markings actually started before that. John had a pinched ear beginning at the age of 3, when his father got sick. Up until that point, he had been extremely close to his father. This was a sign that someone suppressed his behavior; it looked as though he probably had to be quiet and be careful not to bother his father because his father was so sick. John confirmed this. After his father's death, John's mother promptly moved away. She remarried when he was 7, and once again the markings on his ear showed something was taken away from him. But he was adopted by his stepfather and ended up having a close relationship with him. The rest of his childhood was relatively happy. John's mother and stepfather never mentioned his father again. John never even saw a picture of his father and was not allowed to contact his father's family. His father had vanished.

His next big marking occurred when his stepfather died; his ragged hairline showed the trauma in adolescence. His mother died when he was in his early twenties, and it marked heavily across his forehead. John had a lot of loss and grief in his life, and yet he never associated these deaths with his fear of abandonment.

Because John had so many losses in his life, he married early. He marked this event across the middle of his forehead. The bottom of his forehead marked during the divorce that followed 2 years later. After his first wife left, John remarried in his early thirties and had children in his mid-thirties. The lines under his eyes showed the stress involved with raising children, but he was happy and successful in his career. He believed that by having children, he would finally have people in his life who belonged to him and would never leave him. This fear of being left drew that issue back to him, and several years later, his business failed, and his business partner left him. Soon after, John's wife divorced him, took the children, and moved to a different state. These traumas all marked as severe lines across John's nose. His worst fear kept coming true: everyone was always leaving him!

John was a bachelor for most of his forties and worked on rebuilding his career. Finally, in his late forties, he found love again. He desperately wanted to make his relationship last. John was engaged to be married but was terrified of being left. He wanted to know what he needed to do so that his fiancée would not leave him too.

Whenever people confront one of their primal issues, they always need to go back to early childhood. John's abandonment issue stemmed from the death of his father. He was very close to his father and blamed himself when he died. Also, most people don't realize how shut down someone becomes when dying; it takes a lot of energy to die. His father actually abandoned him before his death. So, because of this trauma, he tried to be a good little boy and behave. He did all the right things to please his cranky father but in actuality shut himself down and learned to live "out of his body." He spent the rest of his childhood trying to be the perfect kid so that nothing would happen to his mother or stepfather. Craving love as he did, he still never really let himself receive enough because his fear of losing it prevented him from asking for it.

I asked John to find out about his father, to look for pictures, contact his relatives, and find ways to find out who his father was. He found a picture of his father holding him as a baby and looking at him with intense love. John placed that photo in his wallet to help him remember that he had once been loved that much. John found a way to reconnect with his father. He then went through a period where he resented his mother and stepfather because they took his father's memory away. John had to work on forgiving his mother and stepfather because they did the best they could. They had tried to give him a good life, and he needed to be grateful to them. They were his second and third instances of major abandonment, and he had to process the grief of their deaths too. He needed to realize that they had loved him a lot.

I eventually asked John bring his fiancée in, and she told me about how difficult John was to be in relationship with, even though she loved him. She told me it was impossible to argue with him. Whenever they would have even a small disagreement, he would be terrified that she would leave, so he would avoid confrontation at all costs. If she tried to get him involved in an argument, he would pull away so strongly that she would feel rejected. He would "leave his body." It seemed to her that he didn't care enough to fight for their relationship. She would pull away, which resulted in John pulling away even more because of his fear of rejection. John used to say things like, "Just go ahead and leave!" which was exactly the opposite of what he truly wanted. She couldn't understand why disagreements were such a big deal to him; to her they were a way to clear the air and work things out. For John, it felt like life and death because of his major fear of abandonment.

John needed to stop fearing abandonment so much, and I encouraged him to look at the issue from the deepest level. He was actually leaving everyone else first. He was abandoning his own needs by pulling away in fear. He wouldn't ask for what he wanted, wouldn't explain what was wrong, and would just disappear when people were trying to engage his attention. He was creating a cycle of abandonment.

Ultimately, all issues always come back to the self, and the resistance to future pain and trauma can actually create them. John needed to learn to stay present and ask for what he wanted. He was going to need constant reassurance from his fiancée that she was not leaving him just because they had an argument. He needed be able to reassure himself that he was worthy of being loved. Most important, he had to learn to stay in his body and in the moment.

I heard from John later, after he married. He told me that his heart condition had improved and the tension in his back had lessened so much that he hardly ever took pain medication. His abandonment issue was definitely tied to his health problems, and he had finally taken responsibility for his own happiness. His amygdala probably still overreacts in disagreements, but he knows now how to overcome the panic and fear that arise and has learned to stay connected. The lines and markings on his face indicating the old trauma have lessened, and he looks younger and happier. He is getting the love he has always wanted. I am happy to say that they are still married.

CRITICAL TRANSITIONS

Most childhood issues resurface to be worked on again and again. The first time these issues come up in a big way is in adolescence. This is what the Chinese call the first "critical transition," when childhood issues reemerge as major life lessons to be worked on. This period is shown on the hairline starting at age 14 (Chinese age; 13 in the Western system). In many cultures of the world, this is the time of achieving manhood and womanhood, with ritual ceremonies occurring to mark the shift between childhood and adulthood. Only a few cultures keep this tradition alive. In the Jewish tradition, boys have a *bar mitzvah*, and girls have a *bat mitzvah*. Native Americans have a vision quest ceremony. But in the Western world this transition is mostly ignored, and we suffer the consequences of delayed adulthood.

Most people have irregular hairlines, which indicate the ups and downs of the teenage years. Because most adolescents don't have the time, ability, or interest to resolve their issues, they usually push them down to be dealt with later. They often tend to act out instead of looking in. Childhood issues are the cause of much of the teenage angst that occurs. Unfortunately, most teenagers have not been given very many tools for insight.

Because most people cannot handle this first major critical transition, they wait until the world keeps confronting them with their issues before they start seeing a pattern. Any time I find adolescents recognizing their issues, I rejoice! They are so much likelier to stay healthy and to get focused enough to find their path earlier than most people of the previous generation, including their parents. I've got my sons recognizing their patterns whenever they come up, although they would still rather hang out with their friends than deal with their issues. Try telling a 16-year-old that her boyfriend is a lot like her father. She probably won't believe you and then will promptly get grossed out by the idea. It takes a few repetitions of the pattern before the information starts sinking in and realization occurs.

For most people, the easiest critical transitions to assess are on the face proper from the forehead at age 19 (18 Western), which is the Western milestone for adulthood. The adulthood markings begin just under the hairline and terminate at the chin at age 70. Both men and women have the same age positions down this central meridian, but as on the ears, the markings on the sides of the face are mirror reverse for the different sexes.

I spend most of my time reading the central corridor of energy on the face (Figure 1-4). This line divides the face into the *yin* and *yang*, which we will discuss later. It also is part of the *ren* and *du* channels of the eight extra meridians, which has to do with the sea of *yin* (the kidney *jing*), its use and overuse, and associated issues of fertility and longevity. Any marking across this central corridor or meridian indicates events that are life changing and energy shifting. The stronger the line, the bigger the lesson. Unfinished or partial lines indicate lessons in progress that are incomplete. For example, I had a client who became sober at the age of 27 after many hard-drinking years. But the line was shallow and incomplete across the bottom of his forehead. I concluded that the lesson of sobriety was not fully learned even though it was important. Sure enough, in his late thirties, he had a relapse and another period of serious drinking. He finally learned the lesson thoroughly, as was evidenced by the strong markings under the eyes and renewed sobriety by the age of 39.

This corridor of energy shows when incidents and traumas use up or redirect the *qi*. How well someone has fared in adult life can be easily determined just by looking down the center of the face and evaluating the markings on each feature.

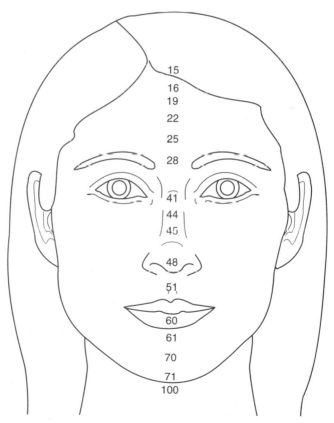

FIGURE 1-4.   Central Corridor of Energy.   Numbers indicate Chinese age. Subtract 1 year for Western age.

Whenever I see heavy markings, I am actually pleased. It means that this person has learned some valuable lessons and has changed because of what has been learned. If the lines are faint, they are probably just repeating a pattern without much consciousness. The stronger the markings, the more thoroughly someone is working out important issues, and the healthier the person will be eventually.

Each feature on this central meridian is approximately 10 years of time, and one of the easiest ways to read the face is to look at the age period as a whole. The forehead is the twenties, the eyebrows and eyes are the thirties, the nose is the forties, the mouth is the fifties, the chin is the sixties, and the jaw is the seventies. Any feature that is clean, even, beautiful, and well marked gives the potential for good luck during that decade.

My grandmother used to tell me to get ready for future luck. She thought nothing was unluckier than not being ready. She always said that when times were bad, it was best to go back to school, travel a lot, or have a baby. All of these things were not considered very lucky because they took such a toll on the body, but they were the best of bad luck (the Chinese have unusual ideas about what luck is!). Then, when the good luck came, you would have your education out of the way, your wanderlust would be spent, or the total responsibility of a small child would diminish some when the child started school. You would be free and ready to do what you were supposed to do.

Any feature that is misshapen, irregular, out of proportion, or distorted can signify a difficult time coming. Let's take the forehead and the twenties as an example. Many stresses occur in the twenties under the guise of having fun. Much overuse of the *jing* occurs too.

I once gave a talk to a group of doctors on April Fool's Day, which I thought was very funny. They were more than a little resistant to the concept of the facial map and skeptical of its validity until I pointed out that nearly everyone in the room had the same kind of deep lines and hollowing on the forehead from the mid- to late twenties. I pointed out the five exceptions and then asked the group what they could have had in common at the period in their lives.

As they looked around the room, and they realized that they all did have very similar markings, a few of them started to laugh. One of them finally yelled out, "Medical school!" It was confirmed that everyone with those markings on their fore-heads had gone to medical school at the same age. Five others had gone either earlier or later and had marked in an entirely different place. After that, they thought the facial map was fascinating and started to accept the concept. The markings on all the doctor's faces indicated that the stress, pressure, and lack of sleep during medical school had taken quite a toll on their *jing*. Their way of thinking about the world was forever altered. They became different people, and their lives were changed because of their experiences.

Of particular importance on the facial map is the transition between the features that are mountains and rivers and the ages that are associated. Everyone marks the milestone that a decade birthday represents. I know many women and men who suffered turning 30 or 40 and agonized over turning 50. In traditional Chinese face reading, the time immediately preceding and following a decade birthday was a time to reflect, reevaluate, and make shifts in the life purpose. Many of these periods have been given names in Western psychology such as "Saturn return," the "midlife crisis," or the "empty nest syndrome."

These fascinating periods are when suppressed material must surface to be worked on. People feel as though they're hit by two-by-fours with issues they have already worked on but obviously have not completely resolved. All those old issues they were sure they were done with rear their ugly heads and make them pay attention to their past.

These times, called *critical transitions,* are when almost everyone questions who they are, why they are here, and if they are happy. I call it the time when the armor cracks and light gets in, or even better, the time when you get to fertilize the seeds for your future! You have been out in the world a while, and the clock has begun ticking in your life. You search for meaning. The challenges that come up make you rethink your priorities. Everything is up for review.

The good news is that the more work you do on yourself during these critical transitions, the healthier you will be later. By going through these transitions fully, you can get a new lease on life. Letting go of old patterns releases energy that was bound up and stuck in the past. I call this new energy "reconstituted *jing.*" The wisdom, or "cosmic water," that you gain from understanding your experiences gives you new energy to face the future. Your *jing* energy will never be what it was, but you do get some of that locked up energy back.

However, having personally gone through a hard critical transition a few years ago, I have to say, it's not fun! Do it anyway. Don't avoid it, and do it thoroughly. It pays off. Each critical transition brings valuable lessons, and the relief you get when it's over is so enjoyable. You often don't even notice that it is over until you wake up one day and realize that you are not suffering any more. In fact, it may have been weeks or even months since you felt so blue, tired, or disappointed. Then you realize you have passed through. It's wonderful when you are done, at least for this round!

The first major critical transition is the late teens and early twenties. This is the very top of the forehead in an area that is usually somewhat rounded. The problem with this transition is that this is the time in life when you think you know everything. You are going to do it so much better than your parents, and after you go through it, you finally realize your parents were not so dumb after all. I have met many twenty-somethings who have said things like, "It's amazing how much my parents really know," with amazement in their voice.

Very few people deal with their issues well here. They are usually too busy being out in the world starting a life of their own. They are in school, starting work, or starting families early. In ancient face reading, this was also considered a karmic time. Whatever karma you were carrying from past lives or from your parents shows up here from out of the blue. This area is called "inheritance," and it carries signs of all the things you have inherited from your family, which includes the lessons you have brought in with you.

Things can happen at this time that make no sense. If it is karmic, you can tell because it feels as if you've been sideswiped. Karma hits you when you least expect it, and you can't figure out why whatever just happened has happened. Totally unprepared, you end up learning invaluable lessons about yourself and gaining big clues that help you to get on what I call your "Golden Path." Lines here mark deeply, and the suffering that occurs with the karmic lessons is usually directly applicable to future work and makes sense only when you find your true calling. Then you have that sudden "Aha!" reaction when your life experiences finally make sense.

Most people do not work on their issues that much during their twenties. They are too busy being surprised and shocked about life and figuring that everything going on is just a fluke or coincidence. The forehead also marks here because of what I call the "Oh my God" syndrome. Everything that surprises or shocks causes the eyebrows to lift and helps reinforce the lines of the lessons. People think they know what marriage is like, but until they do it themselves, they don't really know very much. They may think they know what working is like after coming out of school. Surprise! It usually takes hindsight to understand what it is really like to live in the world.

The next critical transition is at the end of the twenties and the early thirties. This shows up at the bottom of the forehead and often shows heavy indentations when it is a difficult passage. This is often considered a spiritual crisis because this is the age when many of the great religious teachers truly found their calling and mission. In astrology, it is called Saturn return, which implies that the heavy energy of that planet creates hardship and suffering at this transit in life. Because most people have now spent about 10 years out in the world, they have begun to realize the world does not work the way they thought.

Many men become very concerned because they have not become the instant success that they were sure they would be by 30 (although this is changing in the dot.com age), and many women are starting to get very concerned about aging. Their biological clocks start ticking. This is usually a time to reevaluate careers and to take relationships more seriously. Many people get married during this time and start their families. Or, they finally move out of their parents' homes! This is often the end of a very delayed adolescence, and it becomes time to act as an adult. I call this time, "cutting the apron strings for good."

The next critical transition and one of the most important occurs during the late thirties and very early forties. This shows up around the eyes and at the top of the nose. People often agonize over the lines that occur here and do not attribute them at all to the issues they are working on. They are most likely seen as signs of aging that increase their unhappiness. But these lines can lessen when the process is done.

This period is often called the *beginning of the midlife crisis,* a time when a general dissatisfaction and malaise occur. Aging becomes a big factor for both men and women as the skin begins to line more and the body begins to sag more. Gray hairs and extra weight start appearing, and that critical age of 40 is looming fast or has just passed. Weren't you supposed to be something or somebody important by the time you turned 40?

This period involves a lot of issues with self-esteem. Many people have children who are growing fast, and this makes them feel old. Or they are panicking because they don't have any children yet, and it feels like their absolute last chance. I know so many women who get serious baby hunger because biology still controls the reproductive organs. This is a time of many divorces as people try to "find themselves," often in the arms of someone else who isn't all that different from the one they left. Many people realize that their job is just not a career; it is unfulfilling and unrewarding, and they struggle to find a new path.

Many of my clients are this age, the tail end of the baby boomers who had such big hopes and dreams and wanted to change the world. What scares me most is how many of them are using disease as a wake-up call because they have so overused their *jing* and lived so hard only to find as they approach 40 that they are not happy. Their bodies end up betraying their still youthful spirit. They are getting sick with illnesses that used to be reserved for people many years older. I am shocked at the number of people with serious diseases that are showing up in the late thirties and early forties. I am also painfully aware that many of them are also dying far too young because of them.

One of the most important markings in this area is the horizontal line that appears across the bridge of the nose between the eyes. This line is a signal of the need to rejuvenate and occurs at the age of 41 (Chinese, 40 in Western terms). It is a minor spleen/stomach area and indicates the importance of self-nurturing, especially through food and monitoring of blood sugar levels. Most people live off their *jing* as if it were a savings account until they are around 40. Remember how easy it was to stay up all night to cram for finals when you were 20? After 40, it can take 3 days to recover from staying up all night for just one night!

The recovery rate for any kind of abuse to the body is slower after 40, and the body transfers energy from a savings account of *jing* to a checking account of *qi*. What you put in is what you get out. The deeper the line, the more the *jing* has been overused, and the more rejuvenation is required or diseases and disorders of overuse start appearing. The immune system begins to get seriously compromised, and one of the best ways to help it is to eat better and get more nutrients into the body.

This line at 40 across the bridge of the nose can also appear because of a major life shift that many people experience at this age. This is a radical shift, such as moving across the world, getting a divorce after being married for a long time, having a baby, or any number of other life-changing events. The way of life can never be the same because this line crosses the central facial meridian at a very important spot.

The next critical transition occurs at the age of 51 (Chinese, 50 in Western terms). This area is on the groove or philtrum between the nose and upper lip. The groove is symbolic of the reproductive organs and was the original lifeline on the face. According to the ancient Chinese, a long, full, or deep groove indicates the potential for longevity or the ability to have lots of children to take care of you when you are old so you will live longer! Horizontal markings across the philtrum show the transition between fertility and creativity. When a line is present, fertility has been compromised or is no longer possible. Up until the age of 50, reproduction drives the sexual urge for most people. After 50, most women experience menopause, and the testosterone levels in men start to drop. The sex drive diminishes, and this vital sexual force that was used for making babies can now be utilized for creativity.

To the ancient Chinese, having babies was a work of art, and creating works of art was just like conception, pregnancy, and birth. I will never forget looking down at my newborn son and being in awe of the miracle that I had been a part of. He was so beautiful, and I had helped make him. I was so proud of my wonderful baby. Then, only a few years later, my son painted a picture of a hummingbird in school, and as he put it up against the wall, he looked at it with this sense of wonder and said, "Mom, I can't believe I made that. It is so beautiful." It sounded just like what I said when he was born. That made me aware of the connection between fertility and creativity.

It certainly takes much creative energy to raise children. The period that follows is usually about the early fifties and is called "the empty nest syndrome." Many parents grieve heavily over the loss of their babies as they mature into adults and move away. But this is the time of life when you are finally freed from your biology and have the chance to take care of your creativity for your own satisfaction. Raising good people is a great thing, but it is also so important to take care of yourself. I would much rather call this period, "feathering your own nest."

Unfortunately, many people also have to revisit their issues in this critical transition of the early fifties because of the vulnerability they feel about aging. To live longer, the body wants to start purging the things that are suppressing optimal health, and all the old issues return. This time, however, they come with many physical ramifications. Almost everyone at this age gets hit by health concerns that were never problems before.

I know many men facing what I call the "aging jock syndrome" who suffer from all the old sports injuries they had in the past. Knees, shoulders, and elbows give out and require surgery. Arthritis flares, and joints ache. They suffer the loss of their once strong and useful bodies. Men who act out instead of looking in often try to reclaim their youth by becoming latter-day playboys with expensive toys such as boats and cars. At work, they fear layoffs and being fired as never before. They are too close to retirement to take any risks with their jobs, and those who lose their jobs suffer much harm to their egos. At this time in life, the male ego gets hit hard, and the fear of aging makes men run back to whatever made them happy before, or they try to live a life they never had.

Women also grieve the loss of their youthful beauty and former svelte shape as the dreaded "middle-age spread" starts occurring. Hormone function drops drastically with all its repercussions for aging skin and bodies and yet gives reprieve to many of the difficult symptoms that plagued their perimenopause years. Women are a little more likely to look inward, but the fear of being replaced by the younger woman is great. They try to use many external remedies to combat aging, including plastic surgery. They lose their primary roles in life and struggle to find their meaning after children. If they can make the transformation from fertility to creativity, they get a new lease on life. Many women find great joy in their freedom. But regret, disappointment, and lost opportunities can become a strong focus and can lead to bitterness as life turns out not to be the fairytale they once dreamed of. They followed all the rules; why aren't they happy?

This is not an easy critical transition, and one of the most likely hits to occur is the death of parents and peers. This brings up tremendous fear of one's own mortality, and this period is a prime breeding ground for cancer. If people do too much, the area of the upper lip gets heavily marked, and the prescription is to self-nurture if you want these lines to go away. Once again, I cannot stress enough the importance for doing for oneself during this major critical transition of the early fifties.

The critical transition at 61 (Western 60) is much easier for most people. Markings across the upper chin signify a change of life that occurs in the early sixties. This often correlates with retirement. The relief that many people feel on leaving the work force is energizing, and people can finally find time for their hobbies and pleasures. Unfortunately, retirement is also dangerous. Far too many people die within several years of retirement because they feel unproductive and become depressed. They no longer have a reason to get up in the morning and are lost souls.

The key is not to retire but instead to transition to a very busy life doing other, more enjoyable things. Keep working, but have fun! This period also starts easing people into becoming old, and the acceptance of aging is usually more graceful here than the angst so apparent in the fifties. Grandchildren are often a great delight, and people have a chance to make up for their mistakes of parenting with their children's children.

Potential poor health is shown in the sixties by a variety of markings across the chin. Most common are digestive disorders and structural problems with the body such as back pain, broken and brittle bones, and joint problems, as well as problems with memory and forgetfulness. Fear is the primary emotion to be dealt with because courage wanes as physical strength lessens. The right use of will means to stop wasting willpower by trying to make things happen that aren't supposed to.

By their sixties, people are old enough to have gained a lot of wisdom from experience, and one of the most painful things to do is watch their children and grandchildren make similar mistakes and suffer through their issues without listening to the advice of their experienced elders. Yet they are young enough to still play, and that is one if the most important prescriptions. Overall, this is one of the easier transitions, as is the last one in the seventies.

With turning 70, an acceptance of old age comes. This area is shown across both sides of the jaw. Any markings here show potential problems at this time. The second childhood begins here as the face becomes fully marked one time and then starts to mark all over again. Many people at this age need to be cared for and are cared for by their children or are in nursing homes. There is no reason for them not to be vital, but in the Western world, the benefit of a 70-year-old to society is not valued enough.

Simple pleasures need to be enjoyed, especially as disease often starts taking a toll on the body. The easiest way to get through this transition is to come to an understanding of the past and to let go of all negative emotions. This revitalizes the qi. Rekindling ties with estranged loved ones is also very helpful. Unfortunately, many of the controls on behavior have been let go, and the true personalities of people become manifest. Crankiness and irritability are often present, and the absence of pain is often the greatest joy. People start to look backward instead of forward, and that is one of the major signs of old age.

Keeping active, staying creative, being in loving relationships of all kinds, enjoying simple pleasures, letting go of past hurts, and looking to the future are all things that make people live longer and happier lives.

Any time a critical transition brings old hurts and fears up, they need to be dealt with as thoroughly as possible. Avoid suppression of your issues, for the future toll on your body is a high price to pay later. Face your fears, and you will become stronger, healthier, and happier.

If illness or disease strikes, do not take it as a punishment but rather as a lesson. There can be great gifts from the experience of illness. What is the emotional underlay of this disease? How can you track back to the origin of your pattern that helped create this condition? Be gentle on yourself as you unravel the tangled issues of your past. Do not judge yourself; free yourself. Most diseases are just wake-up calls. Answer. The ancient Chinese had a wonderful saying, "Bless every illness that you get because it did not kill you. It is telling you that you were going the wrong way." When you understand your past, you can face your future without burden.

2 / *The Facial Mosaic*

"There are quantities of human beings, but there are many more faces, for each person has several."
RAINER MARIA RILKE, *NOTEBOOKS OF MALTE LAURIDS BRIGGE*

The face can be viewed as a mosaic of many small pieces joined together to create a whole, which can then be divided back into component parts for analysis. The whole, however, is always more than just the parts and is held together by the glue of the individual spirit that resides within the face. The face is both our mask to the outside world and the access to our inner selves, with clues that are readily apparent if we just start noticing them.

The primary way the Chinese divide the face is to look at the two halves. They start with the division of one into two—the *yin* and the *yang* of the face (Figure 2-1). *Yin* and *yang* are interdependent polarities. Neither exists without the other. There are many aspects to these two polarities. *Yin* embodies properties such as cold, feminine, and damp. *Yang* encompasses hot, masculine, and dry. (Box 2-1 lists examples of these functions of *yin* and *yang*.) *Yin* and *yang* have the interesting ability to become the other at any time because each contains the seed of the other. The *yin* and *yang* of the face occur because of the desire to have a public mask and a private persona. What you show to the world is not always how you really feel. This creates the internal/external polarity. If you look at anyone's face very carefully, you can see many subtle differences on the two sides of the face. Learning how to read the two sides gives you access into someone's true nature as opposed to the projection shown to the world (Figure 2-2).

The easiest way to evaluate the two sides of the face is with a photograph. Take a photograph, divide it in half, and look first at one side and then the other. Look carefully for subtle differences in the shape and size of the features and the amount or depth of the lines. You will see a great deal once you start looking. Better yet, scan the photograph and create on a computer a composite of the two right sides of the face versus the two left sides of the face. What you get are two

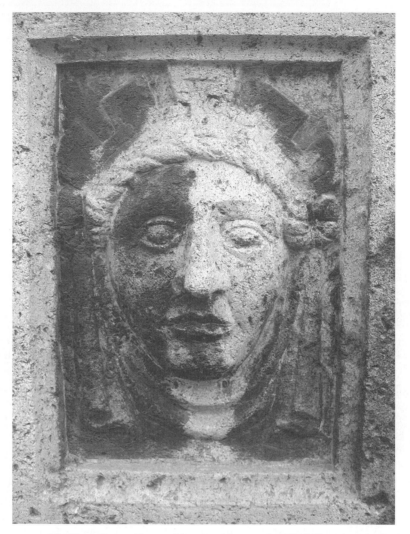

FIGURE 2-1.   *Yin/Yang* Stone Face. After teaching at the TCM Kongress in Rothenburg, Germany last year, I was walking back to my hotel room and was captivated by this *yin/yang* image in stone created by exposure to the elements over time.

different-looking people. You end up with a strange set of twins. The two right sides almost always look a little more pleasant, placid, or calm, whereas the two left sides usually show many more markings and shadows (Figures 2-3 and 2-4).

What do the differences mean? How do the two sides of the face become different? The Chinese have studied this phenomenon for centuries. They consider the right side of the face to be the *yin* side. (This is the individual's right side and is seen by others from their left.) *Yin* is passive and therefore the less emotional side. This is the side that is shown to the world. It is the public mask. Your left side

BOX 2-1   *Yin* and *Yang* Functions

Right Brain	Left Brain
Female	Male
Earth	Heaven
Dark	Light
Cold	Hot
Soft	Hard
Negative Pole	Positive Pole
Feeling	Thinking
Emotional	Logical
Intuitive	Analytical
Creative	Practical
Wholistic	Sequential
Unity	Duality
Reserved	Expressive
Idealistic	Realistic
Passivity	Activity
Parasympathetic Nervous System	Sympathetic Nervous System

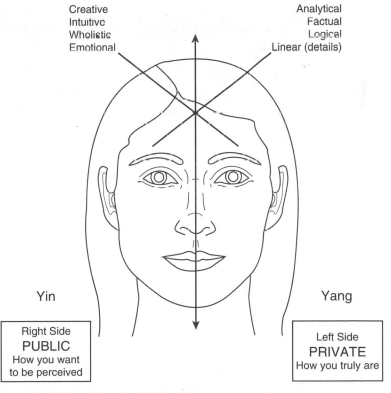

FIGURE 2-2.   The *Yin* and the *Yang* of the Face.

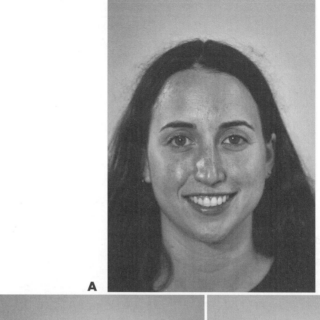

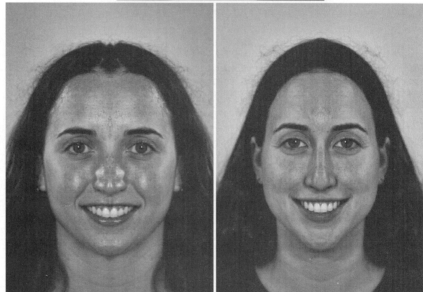

FIGURE 2-3.   Two Sides of the Face—Female.   This lovely young woman appears more social to the outside world because of a wider right side of her face. However, she is more introverted and also happier on the inside, as is seen in the photo of her two left sides.

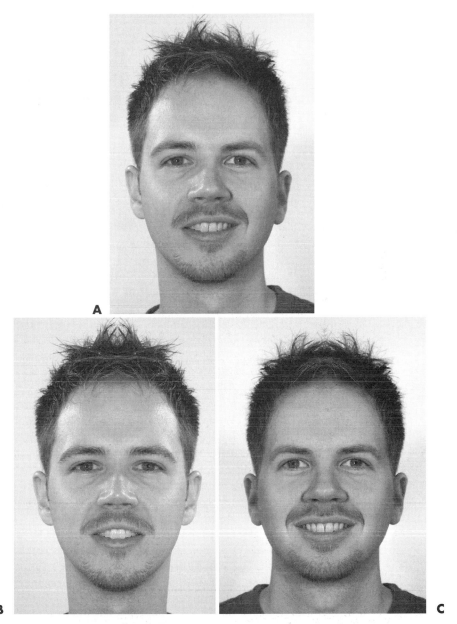

FIGURE 2-4.   Two Sides of the Face—Male.   This handsome young man appears more cerebral and aesthetic from the right side of his face. Based on his two left sides, he is more down to earth and grounded than he seems.

is the more active side and shows more inner emotions, but these have not been expressed publicly. This is the side that holds onto everything repressed.

Western scientists have also studied this phenomenon of facial asymmetry and have discovered it can be linked to split brain function. Both sides of the brain are equally important, and neither side is better than the other. The left side of the brain is logical, factual, detail oriented, and analytical. This side of the brain corresponds to the opposite side of the body. For example, when a stroke occurs in the left hemisphere, it paralyzes the right side of the body. When you are thinking and using the left side of your brain, the corresponding right side of the face makes few expressions and therefore marks less over time. The one exception is the joy lines around the eyes that indicate someone laughs or smiles a lot. These may mark more on the left side because humor is primarily a left-brained function. The juxtaposition of seemingly unrelated things causes surprise, laughter, or amusement.

The right side of the brain is creative, wholistic, intuitive, and emotional. It synthesizes the details the left side of the brain picks up. The right side of the brain feels the emotions and sends them to the left side of the face to be expressed. If it is meant to be publicly expressed, it will go over to the right side within milliseconds. If there is any blockage to expressing, the emotion is pushed down and inhibited. If this repression is a frequent occurrence, the left side becomes more heavily marked over time.

Ideally, both sides of the face should be as symmetrical as possible for optimal health. People like this show how they feel when they feel it. The desire to hide our true nature or our deeper emotions keeps us out of *yin/yang* alignment. Both sides of the brain should be used because they are both necessary for full functioning. In the Western world, we are encouraged and even trained to become left-brain dominant. These traits are simply more valued. Businesses focus on left-brained thinking with the focus on details, the bottom line, organization, and efficiency. Children are encouraged to become more and more left brained as our schools focus on reading, writing, and arithmetic. If school districts have to cut their budgets, they usually eliminate art, music, and physical education—all right-brain–balancing activities.

Luckily, our society is starting to rediscover the value of the right brain. A whole movement has started to help people become more right brained. Doctors have discovered becoming ambidextrous is advantageous to individuals after a stroke. The ambidextrous patient will not be nearly as incapacitated, and recovery occurs quicker. Psychologists are recommending that people start using their nondominant hands and eyes to achieve brain balance.

Another fascinating and related fact about brain function is that men and women use their brains in very different ways. Men use one side of their brain at a time, whereas women can access both sides of the brain at the same time. This is a result of the increased number of connections in the corpus callosum of a woman's brain, a part of the brain scientists have also found to be enlarged in women.[1]

---

[1]Sabbatini RME: Are there differences between the brains of males and females? *Brain Mind* www.epub.org.br/cm/Oct/Dec 2000.

Dr. Bennett A. Shaywitz[2] of the Yale University School of Medicine found women process verbal language on both sides of their brain, whereas men process it on the left side only. This may explain why women's faces get more lined than men's faces: they can think and feel simultaneously.

The markings and lines are heavier and deeper on the left side of the face in individuals who repress the public expression of their emotions; this, like left-brained thinking, is encouraged in our society. Yet most people look only at our passive right masks and rarely even notice the left side of the face. Because more than 80% of the population is right handed, the majority are also right-eye dominant. Because the eyes focus in toward a single point, most people use their dominant right eye to pick up the information on another person's face. Because our brains are lazy, we assume the face is a double right-sided composite. People just don't look at the left side very often unless they are left-eye dominant. I believe these people are getting a much better read on people because they are getting so much more information and are able to synthesize it. You can test your eyes to find out which one is dominant by paying attention to which eye you use when you focus a camera or a pair of binoculars. You can also roll up a piece of paper like a spyglass and put it up to your eye. Which one did you choose? That's your dominant eye.

The bottom line is if you want to get to know someone better, use your left eye, which taps into your right brain, to look at the left side of the person's face and compare it with the right side. You will be amazed at what you see. What exactly do all the differences mean?

Any feature that occurs on both sides of the face can be evaluated. The easiest and most obvious feature to evaluate is the eyes. Most people look at eyes first anyway. The overall size and shape of both eyes is evaluated first, then the reader determines which one is smaller and which is larger.

Eyes are measured in terms of vertical height; how open they are indicates how big they are. Eyes correspond to the heart. If the heart is open, the eyes will be open. If the heart is shut down, the eyes will be narrowed. People who have been badly hurt in the past often have eyes that are held so tightly narrowed they look as if they are squinting. These individuals watch everyone carefully and have major trust issues.

People with large eyes are emotional, expressive, and receptive. Emotions are easily revealed because they are easier to see, and these people are more receptive because they take in more emotional information. If you were to open your eyes very wide while around other people, you would immediately feel very exposed and vulnerable; you are taking everything in. It feels safer to narrow them slightly and watch. Big-eyed people tend to be warmer and more trusting, sometimes too much so.

I once had a student named Karen who had large, beautiful, blue eyes that were so trusting and innocent she looked like a deer caught in the headlights. She was so sweet. She asked me how to find a good relationship because her previous marriage had been very difficult. Karen had married a domineering

---

[2]Shaywitz BA, Shaywitz SE, Pugh KR, et al: Sex differences in the functional organization of the brain for language, *Nature* 373:607-609, 1995.

and emotionally abusive man. Karen was so receptive to my advice it actually made me nervous. I asked her whether she chose men or they chose her. She seemed very surprised at the question. Karen responded that men always chose her and that she was grateful to attract their attention. I told her the best way to find a good man was for her to watch them and that she was the one who was supposed to choose. I told her to start narrowing her eyes and to start watching the men she met. I counseled her not to listen as much to what they said; she needed to watch what they did. I warned her to find a man who was nice to the people in his life: his mother, children, and co-workers. She kept trying to narrow her eyes and couldn't. She had never watched anyone because she was so trusting and believed everyone was good.

It took months of my coaching for Karen to start actually watching and narrowing her eyes, but as summer approached, she was ready. As the next semester started, she came back to inform me she had watched men all summer and she had finally chosen one. She told me he took his mother grocery shopping every week and had a son from a previous marriage whom he treated well and, most important, he was kind to her. Karen had narrowed her eyes to watch and weed out several men who would not have been as good for her.

Eyes that are perpetually held narrowed can also cause difficulties. Narrowing of the eyes shows the heart has been closed or shut down, usually because thinking has taken over feeling. It can also indicate suspicion or lack of trust in others. It is often a sign of previous emotional abuse or a life that has limited feeling. This trait is often tied to heart disease, where an emotional opening of the heart needs to occur for healing. Constantly narrowed eyes indicate people who are analytical and perceiving: people who like to think. Spend a minute trying to solve a math problem and you will notice you automatically narrow your eyes. Thinking makes your eyes smaller.

Eyes are shaped by the constant use of the eyelids. A person may be born with large eyes and hold them narrow because of life experiences. A person with small eyes can hold them open to express and receive as much emotion as possible. What you do with your eyes matters more than what you started with. Because the eyelids are under our control, the best advice is to narrow your eyes when you need to watch and think and open them when you need to feel or receive. Don't get stuck living just one way. Evaluate people by determining whether they are holding their eyes open or narrowed. This is the baseline for receptivity and emotional expression.

Next, look to see which eye is larger than the other. A person whose right eye is bigger than the left eye appears to the outside world to be open, emotional, and receptive, but in reality, on the inside, the person is really analytical, perceiving, or watchful. An individual whose left eye is larger than the right eye is showing the analytical thinker to the world or trying to appear savvy or shrewd. In reality, this is a softy who is receptive, emotional, and expressive in private. This is slightly more common in business people, where it pays to look like a thinker and to hide the feeler.

The next area to look at is the markings around the eyes. The lines around the outside corner are often referred to as "crow's feet." The Chinese call them joy lines. If you have these delightful lines fanning up from your eyes to your forehead, congratulations! If you don't have any, go get some. These lines are formed by constant and repetitive smiling and laughing. Although excess joy is considered a problem in Chinese medicine, I have rarely seen too much happiness! I think a more correct translation would be that excess excitement or manic behavior is dangerous. Smiling and laughing frequently are very positive actions. Many studies show the benefits of smiling and laughing as a method of pain relief. Plus, if you can laugh at yourself and your life, you will be a lot happier. These lines are common on both the right and left sides of the face because people are usually willing to express their happiness and humor.

Unfortunately, these joy lines are paired with the downward set of lines called sadness lines. If these lines radiate over the cheekbones, they become sorrow lines and then grief lines as they pass down into the cheek area. These lines and emotions are much more difficult and tend to be repressed. These emotions are very private and not easily expressed in the world. Therefore they are much more common on the left side of the face. Not only that, but our society does not allow active expression of these emotions. They are not socially acceptable in public.

Lines that start at the outside corner of the eyes and go down toward the nose at a diagonal are called pain lines. Pain is often a very hidden condition. In our society, we encourage people to have a "stiff upper lip" or to "tough it out." Acting stoically to suppress pain is actually counterproductive and increases the pain. The pain becomes intensified even though it is hidden. Chronic pain is not easily shared, and suffering is usually a private affair. Therefore pain lines show up much more on the left side of the face.

Another set of lines starts under the eyes in the inside corner and radiate out under the eye. These are called "lost love" lines. This can be any kind of lost love—a person, pet, job, or way of life. Because this is also private, it will show up more on the left side.

Other features are also very informative when you are evaluating the *yin/yang* balance of the face. The next most expressive feature is the mouth. With the mouth, the most important indicators are the corners. Ideally, both sides of the mouth should turn up. This trait is most easily seen when a person is not smiling. In ancient China, a woman who had a mouth with corners turned up was said to have the "courtesan's smile." Courtesans with this trait were usually favorites with the Emperor because they were so pleasant to be around. It is not actually a smile. It is an energetic upward lift of the corners of the mouth that shows an inner optimism and positive outlook. This emotion of cheerfulness is easily transmittable to others and reflected. The *Mona Lisa* is another great example of how popular this trait is. For many years, people have wondered the reason she is smiling. She is actually not smiling, but the corners of her mouth do turn up, giving that impression. You feel better after having seen this painting; no wonder Napoleon used to hang it over his bed!

On the other hand, down-turned corners of the mouth indicate someone who has been disappointed or who is negative and pessimistic. This is an attitude reflected in the lack of energy it takes to hold the mouth up. Unfortunately, these feelings are a self-fulfilling prophecy. Because these emotions are so contagious, they bring back more negativity.

What does it mean when one side of the mouth turns up but the other side doesn't? People whose right side turns up appear to the world to be happy, but internally, they feel exactly the opposite most of the time. This is like the clown who laughs on the outside but cries on the inside. These people are trying to show the world a positive side, but it is an act. The real self is a disappointed person who suffers alone. When this side is revealed, others are usually quite surprised. This act is perpetuated throughout popular culture, as in the phrase "put on a happy face."

Those whose right sides turn down and left sides turn up are people who expect the best on the inside but prepare for the worst on the outside. They are afraid of showing anyone how much they want something because they will be disappointed if they don't get it. The public pessimist here is really a closet optimist. It is far wiser for these people to show their positive expectations than to hide them. Why would someone hide the happy self? I once had a Japanese client who was not allowed to be cheerful as a child. It was considered unseemly behavior. Her parents valued a serious nature, so she was always scolded whenever she acted positive or optimistic. To this day, she hides her bubbly and playful personality until someone gets to know her. The two sides of her face show this trait clearly.

So how do you get the corners of your mouth to turn up? It takes some time, but cultivating optimism is the first step. This is such a valuable trait. Studies have shown that optimists live longer than pessimists, as much as 19% longer. [3] Optimism is tied to success, good health, and positive outcomes because people expect what they get. Learn to bounce back from disappointments and don't suppress your sad feelings; let them out fully and then think positively. Also, stop smiling when you don't want to. A false smile creates tremendous tension in the face. The expression is forced, not real. If you smile falsely at a dog, it may growl and try to bite you. To a dog, this is an act of baring your teeth and is a sign of anger and aggression. Overusing the facial muscles without the real emotion behind it tires out the muscles. Instead of pretending, find something to laugh and smile about naturally. Cultivate optimism. The corners of your mouth will start moving up before you know it.

Another important area of the face to evaluate for sidedness is the temple area. This area can be hollow or protruding, light or dark. This area shows an individual's "desire for altered states" (see Chapter 4), which is related to liver function.

Because this area indicates the desire to be present, it is also considered or interpreted as one of the indicators of the will to live. It can show whether or not someone wants to live. It is the emotional aspect of the will to live. If both sides are very hollow, it can be a sign of suicidal tendencies. If they are both dark, this person may be using drugs or alcohol as a tool to achieve this self-destruction. Mental illness is also a possibility. When very light, it is a sign of spirituality and creativity.

Another major area associated with the will to live is the cheek area. This area shows the "breath of life" and the functioning of the immune system. The cheek area is involved with the lungs and is a place that shows suffering. When the cheek area beneath the cheekbones and above the jaw is hollow, it indicates overwork, stress, and someone who is going too fast. They are prone to shallow breathing, and

---

[3]Maruta T, Colligan RC, Malinchoc M, Offord KP: Optimists vs. pessimists: survival rate among medical patients over a 30-year period, *Mayo Clin Proc* 75(2):140-143, 2000.

they do not clear out the toxins. If the area is dark, it is a sign that their immune system is toxified, and an illness is imminent or not yet diagnosed. This area is very useful for evaluating a claim of remission, especially if you focus on the left side. Relapse is most easily seen here. People who have hollow or dark cheeks are not really living either. They are merely existing or surviving. To enjoy life fully, an individual has to slow down enough to feel it.

If the temples and cheeks are both hollow and dark, you have the beginnings of the "death mask." This is an unforgettable vision. It appears up to several weeks before death and can come and go for short periods as a person builds up the energy to prepare to die. The face appears cadaverous and looks as though the energy is being sucked out from within it. There is a lack of fat under the skin and an overall darkness in coloration, more like shadows than skin tones. This is believed to be a signal that the soul is leaving the body and is the only sign in face reading of impending death.

The last trait in the will-to-live trilogy is the chin. This is a feature that shows the inherent will of a person in its strength and size. The longer the chin is, the stronger the will. Originally, a long chin was a sign of a longer life, unless, of course, the subject used willfulness to become reckless. The longer chin indicates an ability and willingness to work until the end of life. This purpose contributes to a longer life. This does not mean people with small chins will necessarily die that much younger, but they need to retire and coast until the end of their days. The lack of purpose is the key difference. Chins can also be evaluated for sidedness. A stronger chin on the right side shows a public will but no private will, and a stronger chin on the left side shows a very strong private will in a person who does not force it in public.

Many other traits can be evaluated on the two sides of the face. Eyebrows show temper and an argumentative, driven person. A stronger right eyebrow indicates that a show of anger or drive is easier in public than private. A stronger left eyebrow shows the opposite. A higher eyebrow indicates pride; do they show this inside or outside? A stronger cheekbone predisposes the bearer to bossiness; do they reveal this more at work or at home? Big nostrils indicate someone who spends money or energy easily. Are they really frugal or just pretending to be? A fuller mouth on one side or the other can show hidden or exposed sensuality. A broader face can indicate public or private sociability. A larger jaw can show more determination. Is this shown at home or at work?

Almost any other trait from face reading can be evaluated for sidedness and the public versus private expression of it. Most people show traits to the world that they have been rewarded for showing. It is also common to hold your deeper and darker or vulnerable emotions inside. However, the more balanced the two sides are, the healthier a person is likely to be. It takes much courage to show your real emotions and the depth of your emotions to the world. But ultimately, it is worth it. My grandmother used to say all emotions were good as long as they weren't held in. One of the ways I validate people is that I appreciate and acknowledge people's inner selves, and this helps to bring them out. The *yin/yang* method of face reading is more than fun; it reveals the real person behind the mask.

THE THREE ZONES

Another division of the face gives insight into the decision-making process of individuals. Just as the face can be divided into vertical halves, it can also be divided into horizontal thirds, as shown in Figure 2-5. This classic division of energy in Chinese philosophy symbolizes the separation of heaven, human, and earth. The uppermost zone, which encompasses the forehead, is the heaven zone; the middle zone, which holds the eyebrows, eyes, and nose, is the human zone; and the bottom zone of the mouth, chin, and jaw is the earth zone. People can be categorized based on which zone is the dominant or largest zone. This is a wonderful technique to use in assessing people and is invaluable in business, especially as a sales tool.

These three zones give clues about reaction time to outside stimuli and how people decide to act. The dominant zone is considered the part of the face that is longest along the central meridian. The zone of secondary dominance can enhance or detract from the dominant zone, and the least dominant zone needs to be built up energetically. Because the face continues to lengthen as we age, there is always a chance to create a balanced face. However, when the three zones are all equal, confusion occurs until the person learns what total alignment feels like. Until balanced is achieved, the zone of dominance should be used to make important decisions. It can be used as a strength in the decision-making process.

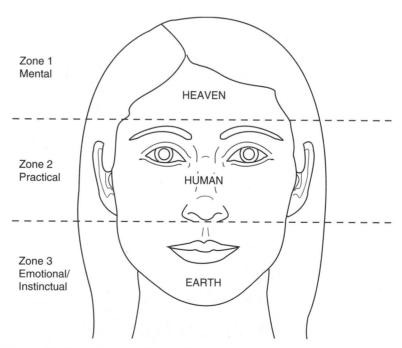

FIGURE 2-5.   The Three Zones of Orientation.   Measure zone 1 from the average hairline to the top of the eyebrow. Measure zone 2 from the top of the eyebrows to the bottom of the nose. Measure zone 3 from the bottom of the nose to the underside of the chin.

The first step in measuring the zones is to evaluate whether any feature on the face is particularly distinctive or larger than the rest. If you can't help but notice someone's large nose or high forehead or long chin, you have already started measuring the zones. The first zone is measured from the average hairline to the top of the eyebrows. A balding man will probably have a dominant first zone (Figure 2-6). If the forehead is also rounded or protruding, this emphasizes the strength of the forehead even more. This is called the mental zone. The forehead is the longest feature on the face and relates to intellect, the mind, and the desire to think things through. People with dominant mental zones are thinkers. It does not mean they are smarter than everyone else, just that they enjoy living in their minds and think all the time. They often have the ability to

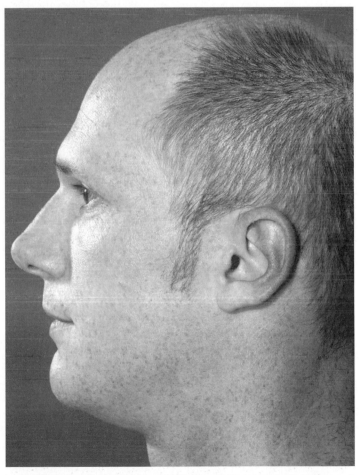

FIGURE 2-6.   Dominant Zone 1.   This is a mental man who thinks a lot before he acts, as seen from his high forehead. The roundness of this feature also shows imagination and a philosophical outlook on life.

overthink, and they rationalize very well. They can be prone to fantasies and fears. When they have decisions to make, they need to spend time thinking and evaluating every option.

Mental zoned people can be indecisive because they want to make the right decision. They love to make "pros and cons" lists. To relate to them better, the best question to ask is, "What do you think about this?" Asking them how they feel is irrelevant because they are thinking! If they aren't given time to think about something, they will say no. They will balk at being forced to make a quick decision. Given a chance, they will research a large purchase. They will read about the item, ask others their opinions, and weigh the good and bad features. Eventually, they will come to a decision but may spend time afterward regretting their decision or rationalizing it.

I had a father with a dominant mental zone, and it took me years to figure out how to handle him. If I wanted to go somewhere, I had to ask him plenty of time in advance. If I rushed him, he would just say no. If I dropped hints, he wouldn't respond until I gave him all the reasons why I should be allowed to go. He still needed time to think about it even after that. His best answer was always, "It's a definite maybe." Finally, right before I needed to go, he usually said yes. It was frustrating for an impatient and emotional child like me, but I learned. I'll never forget that when I wanted to go to college, I was having trouble deciding whether to go to UCLA or UCSB. When I approached my father about my dilemma, his advice was to write a pros and cons list for each school and then make my decision based on which school had more pros. My response was, "But Papa, UCSB is right by the ocean and that counts for a lot!" Needless to say, he didn't get my reasoning and just shook his head in dismay. I ended up going to UCSB first and had a great time. I lived in a dorm room across from the beach. My last year and a half, I transferred to UCLA to graduate.

Zone 2, shown in Figure 2-7, runs from the top of the eyebrows to the bottom of the nose. The nose is the most prominent feature of this zone, which is enhanced by high eyebrows. A nose that is large and protruding or eyebrows that are very thick accentuate this zone even more. The nose has to do with making and managing money and energy. Eyebrows show someone's action orientation, that is, how quick they are to act. People with a dominant middle zone are often business-like and practical and have a lot of common sense. Their sense of efficiency and practicality might not be like anyone else's, but it works for them. To relate to these types better, you might want to ask whether something "works" for them or "makes sense" or "seems practical." This is how they relate to problem solving. They want to save time, money, and energy. They care about how much things cost and love to find bargains. They are not necessarily penny pinchers, but it just doesn't make sense to them to spend more for something they could get cheaper someplace else, unless, of course, they are trying to save time. This is the person who plans trips out of the house with great efficiency. They go to the grocery store after the dry cleaners and the bank because doing the errands this way is much more efficient—the dry cleaners and the bank are on the same street, and the frozen food won't be sitting in the car if they go to the grocery store last. It makes them crazy when someone they live with wastes things, time, or money.

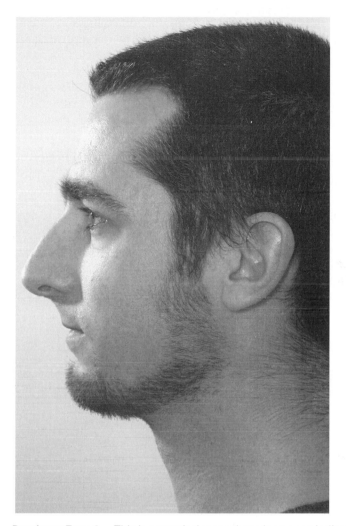

FIGURE 2-7. **Dominant Zone 2.** This is a practical man whose long nose indicates ambition. The dominance of his middle zone shows strong business instincts and the desire to make things work.

This is now my dominant zone and I am getting more and more practical as I get older. I find myself questioning whether I can wait to buy that lipstick when they are giving away those free bonus gifts or watch for when whole chickens are on sale. I don't mind cutting them up, and it saves a lot of money, as deboned chicken breasts cost nearly four times as much. I buy cars that get good gas mileage instead of great looks, although they still have to be attractive enough to suit my sense of style.

One of my students told me a story about being practical that I just loved. She favored champagne-colored cars and Starbucks lattes. She had a little European car, but she spilled her latte every morning and was very frustrated at the stains on the carpet. Because she is a latte addict and must drink it out of the paper cups, she took a full latte to every dealership to test drive the cars! As it turned out, she ended up with an American car because their drink holders were better at holding her lattes. This was a practical consideration for her, but not necessarily for anyone else.

The bottom line is, people with a dominant middle zone are practical and efficient. They save time, energy, and money and want to make things work. They are sensible and function well in the real world.

A long chin makes the bottom third of the face the longest zone (Figure 2-8). Chins have to do with instinct and will. A full or beautiful mouth or a squared jaw adds emphasis to this zone. Dominance in zone 3 indicates people who are

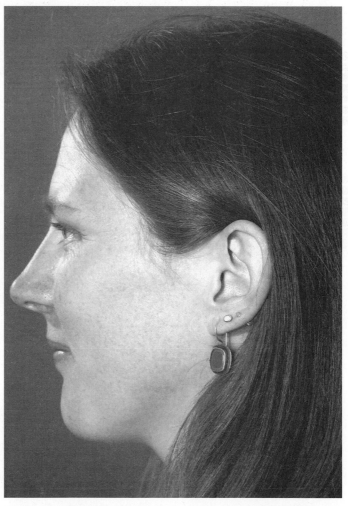

FIGURE 2-8.   Dominant Zone 3.   This is an instinctive woman who can act quickly when it feels right. The fullness of her lips also indicates an emotional nature.

instinctive, willful, emotional, or ruled by their desires and impulses. They tend to do things because they want to or "just have to." They rarely can explain why until later, when they can go back and try to figure it out or justify their behavior. They trust their gut, and they should. They just "know" things. They can be swayed by their emotions and can jump into situations without caution. When asked for a reason, they usually respond that they just had to do it!

Third zone people can scare themselves because they act so quickly, but if they are acting out of instinct, they usually make the right choice. If they act out of emotional impulse, they may find themselves regretting their impulse or even feeling guilty about it, but they still can't help it. To relate better to these individuals, ask them how they "feel" about something, because that's how they operate. These people know what they want when they find it, and then they jump on it. They act before thinking and base their lives on their feelings.

In business, evaluating the zone of dominance is a wonderful tool. Although you need to ask permission before you try to measure someone, it is quite easy to determine a zone of dominance if one feature on a person's face just jumps out at you. If someone's forehead is high and rounded, that's zone 1 dominance. If they have a long nose or big eyebrows, they are most likely zone 2 dominant. If their chin is long and their mouth is generous, you are seeing someone with zone 3 dominance. If any one of these people came to buy something from you, you would sell to them best if you considered their zone of dominance and spoke to them with the right words. By approaching them in the way they operate, they will feel understood and honored.

Let's say you are a car salesman. Salespeople of all kinds are notorious for pitching everything wonderful about their products right away. However, if someone came in who had a high forehead and a dominant zone 1, it would be wiser to relate to the need for information. The person probably has already been researching, which you could discuss. You could also offer any new information the customer doesn't already have. This would be greatly appreciated. These types of customers need to know about the newest technological gadgets and how they work and also about the latest studies. Unless they have completed their research, it is advisable to let them have time to think about it; they will probably come back to buy it from you because you didn't pressure them and were so helpful.

If a person with a middle zone comes to you, you need to get right down to business. This person needs to know such things as how much the monthly payment is going to be—not in an hour, but now. Customers like this will want to know the residual payoff on the lease. They will be inquiring about gas mileage and how far the seats fold down so that their kids can sleep on long trips. They will be fulfilling some need, fixing some problem, or getting a good deal. They worry about data like resale value. This is the important information they require, so give it to them that way. That's how you'll sell them a car.

Zone 3 people are much easier to sell to. If they love it, they'll buy it. The best way to sell the car is to appeal to their emotions. Find the right model and color and take them for a test drive. Ask them to smell the leather seats, listen to the great stereo system, and feel how it handles the road. Tell them how good they look in the car. If these things feel right, you've just sold a car. They are much less concerned about how much the car costs or why it runs so well. They will just love it and have to have it!

Couples usually have different zones of dominance. We tend to marry or connect with people who have what we are missing. When dealing with couples, you need to speak to each of them the way they relate to decision making. And then, you occasionally have a person with balanced zones—what then?

Although balance in Chinese medicine is much valued and is an ultimate goal, having three equal zones is at first difficult. It's difficult because when a decision has to be made, these conflicting desires must line up. Once this is learned, it becomes an invaluable trait. In the meantime, individuals with balanced zones tend to procrastinate because they are waiting for alignment to occur. This takes some practice. What is more common is having two zones of nearly equal value. Then a zone war occurs.

When zone 1 and zone 2 are nearly equal, you have a mental and practical balancing act going on. This requires that plans be thought through thoroughly and then be practical and doable. This is one of the easier balances and is of great help to mechanical engineers and builders. They have vision and planning skills but also have to make things work. Form and function blend well here.

When zones 1 and 3 compete, you have people going through mental and emotional balancing acts. They can spend too much time thinking of things and missing opportunities, or they can jump at things impulsively. What they feel and want is often opposed to what they think. These people can spend large amounts of time justifying things and rationalizing things to make sense of their actions, or they can spend much time inactive because of the fear of making the wrong choice.

Zones 2 and 3 can also be difficult when nearly equal in strength. These people can appear extremely practical and sensible, but that gets boring to them. When they break out and become impulsive or emotional, they kick themselves. I have a zone war like this. Because I get impulsive when shopping for clothes, I have learned to amortize my purchases so that my practical side will be pacified! I have also become an expert at taking vacations at the end of a work trip, which is much more economical.

If one zone is significantly smaller than the others, don't panic. It shows an imbalance but is not a big problem. Having a small upper zone does not mean you lack intelligence. Just don't spend too much time in your head or you will confuse yourself. Don't think too much! Having a small middle zone does not mean you can't be practical or businesslike. These traits just don't come as easily to you and may not be that important. A small bottom zone does not mean you are not emotional. It just means you won't use your instincts or emotions as easily when making an important decision.

My advice is to use your zone of dominance when making an important decision. Use your strength. Go with what you know. Spend other times in your life getting balanced. Ultimately, it would be nice to have all three zones the same, but even then it takes practice to get them all aligned. Also, because the face does get longer as we get older, who knows what you'll be like in the next decade.

FACE SHAPES

Face shapes are one of the most difficult things to evaluate on the face. So many people's faces are a combination of shapes. Face shapes can change very easily over time with weight gains and losses. Face shapes have always fascinated us, particularly in regard to beauty. Many magazine articles talk about what hairstyle each face shape would look good with or what kind of glasses work best. I remember reading an article in *Seventeen* when I was a teenager that recommended I trace my face shape in the mirror with a bar of soap. That was a mess, but I did discover that I had an oval face. My grandfather told me, though, that I had the face of a watermelon seed, which didn't sound that good to me until he told my cousin she had an olive pit face!

Face shapes are the most stereotyped aspect of face reading because they are primarily determined by genetic structure. I view them more as frames for the picture rather than as the picture itself. The traits associated with the individual features carry more weight than the face shape. However, there are generalized traits associated with each face shape that lay the foundation for reading the rest of the face. The shapes are useful indicators of a match to certain professions.

How do you determine face shape? First, look to see whether the face is broad or narrow. The broader the face, the more extroverted the individual appears to be. This correlates with large bones, which show how much physical energy someone has. People with broad faces can tolerate being around other people longer because they have more stamina. It does not mean they are friendlier or more sociable, but, rather that they can handle the company and have the stamina and the energy reserves to deal with others well. People with small bones will have narrower faces. They have less intrinsic physical energy. They may be friendly and sociable but need quiet alone time to recuperate afterward. They absorb others' moods and get drained easily. They have more mental energy than physical energy and work in spurts.

Second, evaluate how much of the face you can see. Are there facial hair or bangs that cover up part of the face? This makes a difference in how an individual is perceived by others. Broader faces are easier to see and therefore to read. The more hidden the face, the less trustworthy people appear to be. In the 1960s, when young men who were hippies had long hair, beards, and moustaches, the establishment distrusted them because they were hidden and therefore considered dangerous. They appeared secretive and scary. The proper look was short hair, so all of the face was easily seen. This is still the norm in the business world.

Third, evaluate the face shape based on three peripheral markers: the temple, cheekbones, and jaw. The width of the face in three areas is measured here and determines the basic face shape (Figure 2-9).

SQUARE

When you look at the square face, the first thing you notice is that it is nearly as wide as it is long (see Color Plate 2). This is a broad face shape. Square-faced people are called "leaders and athletes." These people have strong bones and are

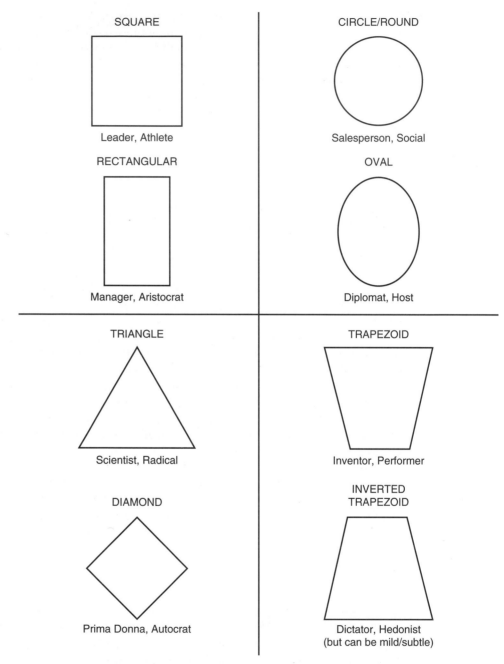

FIGURE 2-9.   **The Basic Outlines of Face Shapes.**

action oriented. Their strong jaws make them more instinctive, so they can often take physical risks because they know their physical boundaries. They are recognized for their physical strength and stamina. They like to have their own way, to be in charge, and to not be challenged. They can be stubborn and willful. They can also be determined and persistent. They have a "follow me" attitude. The squared jaw adds the elements of loyalty and an adherence to principles. You will find this face shape most often in contact sports such as football and wrestling; you'll see it in the police force and in the military.

One of the best examples is Winston Churchill, with his bulldog jaw. He came to power in a time of crisis and led very effectively during the war. He was not as successful in the peacetime that followed. Jacqueline Kennedy Onassis is another good example of a woman with this face shape. This shape is less common in women, and when you do find it, you have a woman who is powerful, athletic, and most likely a businesswoman.

RECTANGLE OR OBLONG

The rectangular face shape shares some traits with the square face, but the face is longer and narrower, so the traits have been subdued. This face shape is a refinement of the square. The temples, cheekbones, and jaw line are still relatively equal, as shown in Color Plate 3. These people are called the *managers* or *aristocrats*. This is the most common face shape in politics and business. Traditionally, it has also been the favored shape in the royal families, and women were sought after who could breed sons with this face.

People with rectangular faces are more idealistic and far sighted. They usually think before they act, although they can act quickly once their minds are made up. They can be authoritative and can inspire confidence. They make excellent mentors and like to help others achieve their goals.

Many presidents of countries, businesses, and organizations have this face shape. These people get promoted to management positions even when they don't seek a leadership role because they look like thoughtful leaders. Good examples are Ronald Reagan, who looked like a president, and Grace Kelly, who looked like a princess. She was the epitome of the beautiful and classic rectangular face shape. This is also the "leading man" face shape, the strong and silent type.

ROUND

The round face is the most trusted face shape. People with this face shape have very broad cheekbones with fleshy pads on their cheeks (see Color Plate 4). It is often associated with weight gain, but it is not always correlated. They are called the *salespeople* or the *partiers*. Their darling chubby cheeks make you want to pinch them, and they always have a look of innocence and childlike honesty. This is the face shape most seen in the good cartoon characters. They are cute, cuddly, and have round features. People with round faces just appear friendly and open. They may actually have forceful personalities behind their friendliness. They can be vigorous and impulsive. They are fond of their comforts and enjoy boisterous behavior. The larger the features, the more ambition you will find behind the round face. Smaller features on a round face indicate an amiable, easygoing nature with less drive. Mickey Rooney is a good example of a round-faced person. I have never heard him criticized for marrying so many times, and he has a boyish charm that makes him very likable. Oprah Winfrey is another example of a much loved and trusted round-faced person.

OVAL

The oval face shape shares many characteristics with the round face, but the face is narrower and more delicate, and the traits become refined, as in Color Plate 5. They are also very social types but are much less outgoing. They are charming and gracious and are the consummate "host" or "diplomat." The oval hairline indicates a strong mother's influence or heavy social conditioning. They are very sensitive and aware of other people's feelings and needs. They want everyone to get along and dislike conflict. They cater to others and can seemingly agree with other people's opinions while holding quite a different personal view that they do not express for fear of offending someone. They value peace and cooperation. They are often well versed in the social graces, have excellent manners, and delegate well. They are usually criticized when they don't act perfectly. It is always such a surprise to find imperfections in these people because they usually look so put together. They often get involved in charitable causes and truly enjoy the fundraising parties.

An excellent example is General and President Dwight Eisenhower, who as a general in World War II was probably the only man who could get all those square- and rectangular-faced generals to work together. Many of the great beauties of Hollywood had this face shape. Elizabeth Taylor is a good example, and her involvement in the AIDS charities shows the tendencies of an oval-faced person.

TRIANGLE

The triangular face shape is characterized by a high, wide forehead, which narrows down to a pointed chin. The face is often considered bony because there is little extra padding on the cheeks, the nose is thin, and the cheekbones often protrude (see Color Plate 6). These people have been named the *scientists* and the *radicals*. They have strong mental ability and focus. These people are introverted and drawn to serious study, intellectual pursuits, and radical ideas. They can be very individualistic and dislike being given orders. Research is often a good field because of their innate ability to organize their thoughts in a systematic way. They often have critical minds and sharp tongues. Unusual ideas or causes can interest these people, and they can be very intense about their beliefs. There may be a danger that they can take things to an extreme and get behind radical causes. However, many triangular-faced people can also be attracted to philosophy and the arts.

My favorite example is Fred Astaire. He was very mental, especially for a dancer, and he choreographed every single dance step in his head before his feet even touched the floor. Albert Einstein had a broad version of this face shape. Timothy McVeigh is an example of the radical.

TRAPEZOID

The trapezoid face shape is similar to the triangle; the forehead is still large, but the face is broader, and the chin is blunted to a rounded or squared shape, as shown in Color Plate 7. Trapezoid people are more sociable than their triangular counterparts, and they take their ideas and bring them into reality. They are known as the *inventors* and *performers*. This face shape is the most common in engineering and the performing arts. The entire entertainment world is full of trapezoids. It is an industry where imagination is made manifest. It is based on make-believe and invention. The trapezoidal types are thinkers who need to do something tangible with their thoughts. They are the inventors who also need to manufacture. People with this face shape enjoy problem solving and brainstorming and the act of creation and building.

My favorite example of a trapezoid is Walt Disney. He had an incredible imagination and founded an entire industry of theme parks. Disneyland is a monument to his creative genius. There are also great numbers of actors with this face shape, from Katherine Hepburn to Kevin Costner.

INVERTED TRAPEZOID

The inverted trapezoid shape belongs to domineering and controlling people. It is called the *dictator* and the *hedonist*. These people love to have power over others—they need it. They are also drawn to material and physical excess and pleasure. Intellectual pursuits are rarely fulfilling; instead, their lives are geared toward achieving dominion over others and vindicating themselves from the perceived mistreatment they received from anyone who stood in their way in the past. They are prone to resentment and have feelings of entitlement. They can be very selfish in their desires and can use strong-arm tactics and bribery as methods of persuasion.

A good example of an inverted trapezoid would be Idi Amin. He banned books and burned them because he didn't read. He had professors killed at the university because he thought they were laughing at him. He had his toilets gold-plated while his people were starving in the streets. Many other dictators in the world approach this face shape as evidenced by the growth of their heavy jowls. But, luckily, most of them started out with other face shapes and have some other moderating features that keep them from being a full inverted trapezoid. Examples include Mussolini, who was originally an oval, Stalin, who was square, and Saddam Hussein, who used to be rectangular.

As scary as this face shape can be, there are many people in the world who develop this face shape and are good people and don't take it to the extremes of the dictator. However, they usually have strong needs to control their family members or their employees, or they are involved with the serious pursuit of pleasure. One woman I knew would not take phone calls until after 11 a.m. because her beauty sleep was the most important thing to her. She would change her plans frequently based on what she thought would be most fun regardless of her previous commitment and always had to buy the best clothing labels, eat at the trendiest restaurants, and be seen with the most popular people. She controlled those around her through her self-centeredness. Another woman I knew with this face shape made her son, who was built like a linebacker, take ballet lessons because she didn't approve of sports.

DIAMOND

The diamond face shape is more common in women than in men and is recognized by broad cheekbones combined with a narrowed forehead and a narrow chin. This used to be called a heart-shaped face. This face shape belongs to people who are called *autocrats* and *prima donnas*. They are high-strung and temperamental people who demand to have things their way. There is an authority with charm that usually guarantees their success at achieving their goals. They can be aggravating and exasperating but are easily forgiven because of their passion and ability to compliment those who do what they want. They have very high standards that border on perfectionism and are absolutely the best at stamping their feet or acting superior.

Maria Callas is the best example of this face shape. Her tantrums were legendary, but so were her talent, charm, and passion.

CHANGING FACE SHAPES

Face shapes can be deceiving because they can change so easily with weight gain and loss. The most important thing to look at is the original bone structure and then evaluate how much the flesh is adding or subtracting from that structure. Some people have combinations of face shapes such as oval on top and rectangular on the bottom. In this case, you combine the meanings of these two types; strong socialization and good manners may be associated with management abilities. The need to please could be holding them back from becoming true rectangles. Perhaps if they expanded their thinking and lost some of their fear, they would have more success in business.

The original face shape based on bone structure is always most important and takes precedence in reading face shapes. As people change their roles in life, their faces will change too. When you run across a combination face shape, you have probably found a person in transition.

To make determining face shapes simpler, remember that if there is a square jaw, you have probably found a square or rectangle. Just determine whether the face is broad or narrow. If you don't see plump cheeks, the person is not round. For an oval, you must have the oval hairline, and the triangle must have the narrow chin with the wide forehead.

There is no ideal face shape. They all have benefits and positive attributes. Although certain professions seem to attract certain face shapes, do not be alarmed if you are different. Every group of like-minded people needs to be shaken up once in a while by someone who thinks or acts differently. And remember, the face shape is just the picture frame. Read the features to find the picture.

The Five Elements of the Face

"The number five represents the five senses, five elements, five colors, five tastes, and the five systems of the body. When the heart is in harmony with the five senses, it is aware. This leads to realization."
ED YOUNG, *VOICES OF THE HEART*

The ancient Chinese used the system of the five elements to divide the world into vibrational families. They discovered that things with similar attributes could be grouped together into archetypal associations with the natural world: water, wood, fire, earth, and metal (also known as air). This five-element system not only described the principal energies of each major grouping, it could also be broken down into smaller subsystems such as the seasons, tastes, colors, shapes, sounds, activities, textures, etc.

The five-element theory involves both the generative and destructive cycles (Figure II-1). These elements can help and harm each other. The generative cycle occurs when water feeds wood and makes it grow, wood becomes fuel for fire, fire creates ash to feed the earth, and earth grows metal, which in turn melts and becomes water. The destructive cycle acts much the same way as the childhood game "rock, paper, scissors." Water puts out fire, wood depletes the earth, fire melts metal, earth blocks water's flow, and metal cuts wood.

Although these elements are easily balanced in the natural world, it becomes an art to balance them in our lives. These five elements are also represented within our bodies as the five major organs and their associated body parts, emotions, and actions (Table II-1). Everyone has all five major organs: the kidneys, associated with water; the liver, wood; the heart, fire; the spleen/stomach, earth; and the lungs, metal. Without these organs, we would die. Because everyone has all five organs, we all have the five elements as part of us. The individual balance of these five elements depends on the functioning and predisposition of each organ and its strength or weakness along with overuse or underuse.

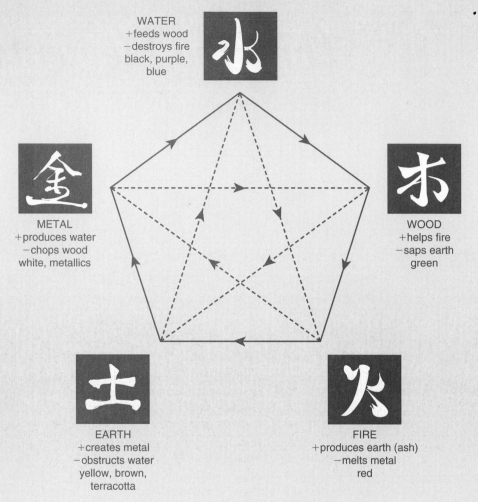

FIGURE II-1.   The Five-Element Creative and Destructive Cycles.

Even the face can be divided into groupings of five element features and their corresponding emotions. These features correlate directly to the organs within the body and indicate their health and functioning. Strength in certain features indicates strength in the related organ and the ability to express the primary emotion that organ controls. Analyzing these features makes it easy to create a snapshot of the inherent personality of someone and an elemental profile. The traits associated with each feature are neither good nor bad; it only matters how they are used. Creating a comprehensive profile is also more important than focussing on the meaning of any individual trait.

However, in analyzing the facial features, the parts must be broken down before the whole can be synthesized. So, let's take a look at the five elements, starting with the water element, from which all life comes.

TABLE II-1   The Five Elements: The Physical Aspects

	水	木	火	土	金
	Water	**Wood**	**Fire**	**Earth**	**Metal**
Organs	Kidney	Liver	Heart	Stomach	Lungs
Body parts influenced	Low back Knees Brain	Tendons Neck Head	Hands Chest Ribs	Spleen Pancreas Muscles Midback	Skin Body hair Upper back Shoulders

Body type	Shadowed eyes
	Big bones
	Wide hips
		Tall/sinewy
		Short/energetic
			Small
			Narrow hips
			Redness or
			   flush in neck
				Rounded
				Fleshy
				Plumpness
					Small boned
					Fair skinned
					Aquiline
					   features

Correlating facial features	Ears Forehead Chin	Eyebrows Browbones Jaw	Eyes Lines Tips/corners	Mouth Lower cheeks Above lips	Nose Cheekbones Moles
Needs	Being Water Time alone Creativity	Doing Trees, plants Focus Intensity	Playing Color Light, heat Talking	Family and friends Comfort Things	Order Purity Boundaries Space and time
Colors	Black Blue	Green	Red, pink Orange	Brown, yellow Earthtones	White, pastels Metal, pale gray
Shapes	Amorphous Curved	Tall Columns Rectangles	Angles Sharpness Corners	Low/heavy Permanent Stable	Round Square Open
Seasons	Winter	Spring	Early summer	Late summer	Fall
Weather	Cold	Wind	Heat	Damp	Dryness
Sound	Moan	Shout	Laughter	Singing	Crying Weeping
Action	Shivering	Clenched fist	Anxious look	Spitting	Cough
Senses	Hearing	Seeing	Feeling	Tasting	Smelling

THE WATER ELEMENT

Water is the most generative force in nature and is what drives the fundamental desire to procreate. This element is symbolized by the seeds that sprout underground in the winter, patiently waiting for their time to emerge. Then, water continues to feed these plants as they grow. Water carves the land with infinite tenacity and perseverance and gives it shape. It is strong, deep, and mysterious.

It is associated with darkness and the colors black and blue. Water is the giver of life on our planet.

Although most of Chinese medical texts focus on wood as the first element of the five-element system, I was taught and have always believed that water was the starting place. We live our first 9 months in a gentle bath of amniotic fluid, and the kidneys are the first organ to be developed *in utero*. Hearing, which is associated with the kidneys, is the first sense to be activated in the womb. Water is about "being," allowing enough stillness to "be," and the ability to let come what will or to go with the flow. It is about getting ready for action.

Our fundamental need for water is made evident in the makeup of the human body, which is composed of nearly 90% water. According to Chinese medicine, the water system of the body includes first the kidneys, then the brain, bones, bone marrow, spinal cord, reproductive organs, bladder, the lower back, hips, knees, teeth, and hair on the head and pubic area. The water system is responsible for the fundamental inherited *qi* called *jing*, which is the battery of the body and the inheritance from our ancestors. Overuse of this system causes aging, whereas wise use and care allow for regeneration. Many signs on the face indicate how strong the water element is, how well the kidneys are currently functioning, and the potential for longevity.

Emotionally, the water element is responsible for fear. This is a powerful and primal emotion that we are confronted with our entire lives. It is the emotion that robs the kidneys of energy when overused and causes dangerous recklessness when underused.

On the face, features associated with the water element can be evaluated for size and strength. The larger or stronger the feature is, the more physical or emotional water strength a person has. The feature that most clearly represents the water element is the ears; this is considered the vital element of the kidneys. After that, you can evaluate the hairline, upper forehead, the under-eye area, the groove or philtrum, and the chin. Each of these features shows either a strength or deficiency in the water element, and together they create a profile of how "watery" a person is (see Color Plate 8).

THE WOOD ELEMENT

Wood is the element of dynamic change and growth. Like the tree it symbolizes, wood rises upward from the ground and is the connection between earth and heaven. The wood element is forceful, strong, and direct. Trees give our planet the oxygen we need to breathe, the shade under which we find protection, and the materials with which to build our shelters. Wood created our first weapons and shields and is symbolized by the warrior.

In Chinese medicine, the wood element is the season of spring and the color green, which symbolizes the new life that emerges and bursts forth from the mysterious inner world to make a mark on the outer world. The wood element corresponds to the liver and is responsible for the emotion of anger and the action of drive. People with strong wood energy love a good fight. This element fuels people to have the energy that helps them go out and conquer the world through work or war. Wood energy is responsible for the ability to push through obstacles and accomplish goals. It is about focus. The wood element is involved with "doing" and "getting things done."

The wood element features show how strong the liver is and how well it is functioning as one of the most powerful internal detoxifiers. The wood system of the body correlates to the gallbladder, the neck and head, the tendons and ligaments, the iris, the sexual organs, and the nails. The vital feature corresponding to the liver is the eyebrows. Strong eyebrows show how much energy and passion a person has to challenge the world. After that, the brow bones, the temple area, the "seat of the stamp," the set of the eyes, the sclera, and the jaw can be evaluated for size and strength. Together, these features can be combined to show how "woody" someone is (see Color Plate 9).

THE FIRE ELEMENT

Fire is vibrant, magnetic, and alive. It stimulates the spirit and excites the mind with dancing flames. Fire is the primal element that lit up the darkness of night and protected us against the unknown. It kept away the wild animals and extended the hours we could stay awake. It was the element to make music by, to dance around, and to sleep near. It created a whole new way of cooking and eating and expanded the ability to explore the world to find new places to live. Fire can be out of control, as a raging wildfire, or tamed in a fireplace or candle. In either case, fire can mesmerize.

Fire is the element of fun and play. It is adaptable and quick to change. Fire rules the heart and the emotion of excitement, usually mistranslated as joy. Excitement, like fire, is temporary and burns out as soon as it loses its source of fuel. Fire constantly seeks new places to burn, just as people with strong fire energy seek new experiences or contacts. Fire is easily extinguished and easily rekindled, as long as there are smoldering embers!

Fire is associated with early summer and the blooming of flowers. Fire is about performance, play, and living in technicolor. The color red and all bright colors show how the fire element attracts attention.

The fire element rules the heart. The parts of the body that belong to the fire element include the small intestines, the arteries, the hands, the chest and ribs, the tongue, and the blood. The vital feature is the eyes. Fire is responsible for the light in the eye, the *shen*. This brightness shows the workings of the mind and the subtle shifts of all momentary emotions. The heart is the emperor of the body and rules over the expression of all other emotions. Therefore the fire element is also seen in the tips and corners of every other feature. All wrinkles and their associated past feelings are associated with fire, even when they are in a part of the face that corresponds to another organ. Fire controls the activity of the brain, the firing of neurons, and the imagination and ideas this creates. The ancient Chinese had a fear of fire because even though fire gives us the zest to enjoy life, it can also wear us out. Fiery people are easy to spot (see Color Plate 10). They have bright eyes, big smiles, freckles, sharp corners to their features, and usually lots of lines showing you how much they can express their zest for life.

THE EARTH ELEMENT

Earth as an element is warm and nurturing. Worshipped as the nurturing "mother" since the beginning of time, earth is the ultimate parent, and all living things are her children. The earth is comforting and calm, solid and stable. Earth stays much the same for centuries. It is the most constant element.

Earth energy is grounding and stabilizing. It is associated with the season of late summer and the harvest. It is reminiscent of the trees heavy with ripe fruit and the lazy hot days where life moves slowly. Earth is about family, community, and gathering. It is about eating now and holding and storing for later. Like the sticky juice of ripe fruit, people with earth energy stay attached to other people, things, and places. Earth is about savoring the sweetness of life and enjoying all of the comforts.

In Chinese medicine, the earth element is about ingestion and absorption. It allows people to take in food or ideas. The organ most closely associated with earth is the spleen/stomach and the digestive system of the body. It also is responsible for the pancreas, the large muscles, the midback, the lymph system, and the diaphragm. Earth element problems in the body often involve stagnation and the slowing down of *qi* or the inability to ingest or digest ideas or food.

The emotions of earth are sympathy or worry, which keep people feeling connected. Its vital feature is the mouth and lips, but it is also associated with the bridge of the nose, the eyelids, and the lower cheeks. The earth element is responsible for all the warehouses or fleshy parts of the face and the ability to hold onto people, things, ideas, or money. People with strong earth energy features know how to relish the comforts of life and the pleasures of being human. There is a fleshy quality to their skin and a softness to their features that show how "earthy" they are (see Color Plate 11).

THE METAL ELEMENT

Metal is the element that is cool, reflective, and unknowable. It can be a pure, rare, and refined substance, like gold, or a composite made up of other metals, like brass. Like the sword, metal can be tempered and strong, and like jewelry, it can be delicate and beautiful. It is a substance found in raw form but is most valued when molded, shaped, and crafted into something unique.

Metal in Chinese medicine is a confusing element and is often given attributes that are less than flattering. The confusion lies in the dual nature of the element. The oldest symbol for metal was the Chinese coin. Not only did it contain two different types and colors of metal, it was also a solid round object with a square hole in the middle indicating air. The duality of the metal element is part of its magic. Like a Zen koan, metal is a paradox and symbolizes everything and nothing, great wealth and utter simplicity, lofty ideals and petty details. Metal values the glamor and graciousness of the past yet values the technology of the future. The metal element is complicated yet ultimately easy to understand.

Metal is associated with the fall and the time when the world is retreating to essence in preparation for winter. It is contraction, and yet it can also be a time of expansion seen in the last brief show of color in the leaves. It is the color white, which is the Chinese color for death, and also all metal tones such as gold, copper, brass, and steel. It is the emotion of sorrow that turns to grief for what used to be or what could have been or what will never be. Metal is about striving for perfection and suffering when it is not achieved.

The metal element is responsible for the lungs, which connect or protect an individual from the outside world. The metal element represents boundaries and taking in or cutting off input. The metal element also controls the upper back, the shoulders, the colon, the sinuses, the bronchi, the mucous membranes, and body hair. The vital feature is the nose, and the corollary features are the underbrow area, the cheekbones and cheeks, and the skin. Look for refined features, a long aquiline nose, a symmetrical face, and delicacy of the bone structure. Fairness and thinness of skin are also good indicators of how "metallic" someone is (see Color Plate 12).

FIVE-ELEMENT PROFILING

To create a five-element profile, the features on the face must be evaluated for size and strength. If the majority of water features on the face are prominent or large, an individual has a lot of water energy. This can be strength in the water element either physically, emotionally, or both. This person's kidneys may be very healthy, or there may be a lot of courage, stubbornness, or will present. If all of the water features are small, there is most likely a deficiency in the water element and probably more fear. Most important, the features must be examined as a group. A person with a smaller feature in one elemental group has an intrinsic balance because of another feature that has strength.

This is true for all of the five-element feature groups. Evaluate each feature of a group individually and then look at the entire set of features to determine the strength or deficiency. The important thing is to look for each person's intrinsic balance. There may be lovely features and beautiful faces, but no face is perfectly balanced. Each face has a unique story to tell about the person to whom it belongs. We'll look first at the emotional traits of the features that tell us about personality and later discuss the health indicators of the face.

3 / *The Water Features and Traits*

"Water, gentlemen, is the one substance from which earth can conceal nothing. It sucks out its innermost secrets and brings them to our very lips."
JEAN GIRAUDOUX, *THE MADWOMAN OF CHAILLOT*

Every feature that corresponds to the water element indicates the physical or emotional strength or weakness of the kidneys and the associated parts of the body. These features show genetic predispositions and inherited or developed personality traits such as courage, will, and stubbornness. Ears are considered the vital feature of the kidneys and are most closely associated with its fundamental *qi* or *jing*.

EARS

First we will look at the inherited constitution. Grasp the ear between your thumb and forefinger and bend the ear forward. Evaluate the strength of the cartilage. Firm ears indicate strength in the kidneys and a healthy constitution. They are indicative of good *jing*. They should not be too stiff, however. The best ears are flexible but have some tensile strength, like *al dente* pasta. Ears that are too stiff indicate a propensity to high blood pressure, and ears that are too flimsy, thin, or transparent belong to people with weak constitutions. The flimsier the ear's cartilage, the more delicate the basic constitution. One of my students showed me how he could fold up his ear into a little package. It was quite alarming. It also indicated how fragile his health was and how careful he needed to be about his lifestyle choices.

The quality of the cartilage of the ear was originally used as one of the predictors of long life. Generally, the ancient Chinese believed that the stronger the ears were, the longer someone would live. Unfortunately, many people with strong inherited constitutions use up or wear out their gift of good health and are struck down by an illness or accident that could have been prevented with wiser management of the *jing*. I call this "*jing* blowout." On the other hand, many people who were born with weak constitutions watch their energy expenditure, guard their health wisely, and end up living to be older than expected. Good use of *jing* is one of the most important determiners of longevity.

The size of one's ears indicates courage or risk-taking ability. Large ears often belong to gamblers. Just walk by the high-stakes poker games in Las Vegas. I have yet to see a serious gambler there with small ears. This kind of risk-taking ability goes beyond gambling with money. Others with this trait feel comfortable gambling with their bodies and sometimes their lives, performing dangerous stunts or having dangerous occupations. They feel that they have the ability to recover from accident or injury easily and exhibit a surprising lack of fear and a powerful belief in their physical abilities. An example of large ears can be seen in Figure 3-1.

Small ears belong to cautious and careful people (Figure 3-2). The Chinese say that children with small ears are very well behaved. They worry about doing something that would displease their parents. Small ears can also indicate a constitutional water deficiency, because these people feel fear very easily. They rarely take risks unless they are very calculated and prefer to live safely, usually by the rules.

The widths across the three different parts of the ear show what kind of risks people are most comfortable taking. People with ears that are broad across the top (Figure 3-3) are capable of taking a mental or financial risk. They would be good candidates for running their own businesses. They don't have to know from where the next paycheck is coming. They are comfortable risking money and don't need

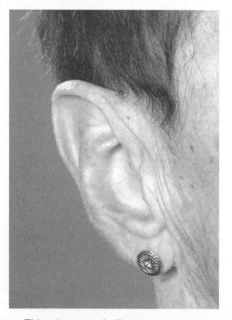

FIGURE 3-1.   Large Ears.   This photograph illustrates a large ear, indicative of risk-taking ability.

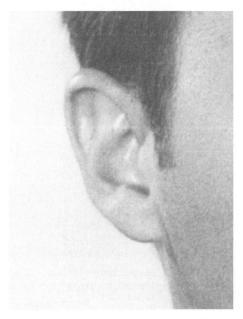

FIGURE 3-2.   **Small Ears.**   This photograph illustrates a small ear, which implies a cautious nature.

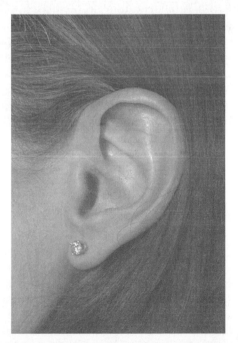

FIGURE 3-3.   **Ears Broad Across the Top.**   The subject in this photograph has an ear that is broad across the top, which indicates the ability to take financial risks.

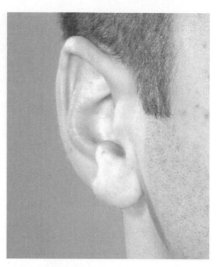

FIGURE 3-4.   Ears Narrow Across the Top.   The subject in this photograph has an ear that is narrow across the top, which is a sign of security issues and the need for a regular income.

as much financial security. Narrowness across the top of the ear (Figure 3-4) indicates a security issue. These people do much better with a steady job and a regular paycheck.

Breadth across the middle of the ear (Figure 3-5) indicates a person who is capable of taking physical risks. These people jump out of airplanes, climb into caves, race cars, or mountain bike down steep inclines. They enjoy testing their physical boundaries and feel exhilarated rather than fearful. People with a narrower area here (Figure 3-6) are very unlikely to do these types of things unless there is a guarantee of safety, such as with rock climbing in a harness. I have narrow ears across the middle, and I personally think camping is a physical risk!

Large earlobes (Figure 3-7) belong to people who are wise and plan for their future, which helps ensure that they have one. They cultivate faith instead of fear. People with large earlobes have the ability to grow things—people, plants, animals, or investments. These people are patient, can delay gratification for future payoff, and have amazing luck with long-term investments such as real estate. Large earlobes are also a sign of being taken care of in old age or having good luck in old age because of good planning.

People with small earlobes (Figure 3-8) tend to live in the present and do not focus on their future. They are interested in instant gratification and do not plan very far. They want to live for now, not later. These people are often playing catch-up when they get to retirement age and probably didn't believe that they were ever going to get there.

Attached earlobes (Figure 3-9) are a sign of a person who is very attached to the family into which he or she was born. This can be a negative attachment if the individual doesn't like or even hates the birth family, but the attachment exists

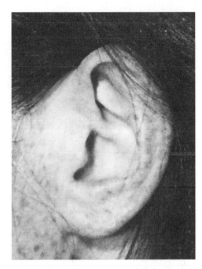

FIGURE 3-5. Ears Broad Across the Middle. The subject in this photograph has an ear that is broad across the middle, indicating the ability and desire to take physical risks.

nonetheless. These individuals have more trouble moving away from them physically or shedding their influence psychologically.

People with detached earlobes (Figure 3-10) are usually attached to fewer members of their immediate family and are more prone to move away or feel indifferent about the rest of their family. They are likely to create friendships that feel like family, including having their children call good friends "Auntie" or "Uncle."

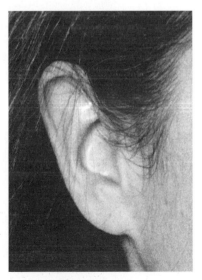

FIGURE 3-6. Ears Narrow Across the Middle. The subject in this photograph has an ear that is narrow across the middle, showing that physical risks are not desired. She requires physical safety.

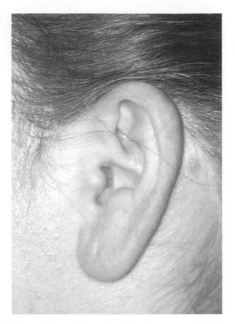

FIGURE 3-7.   Large Earlobes.   The subject in this photograph is future oriented, as is shown by her large earlobe. This is a sign of luck in old age.

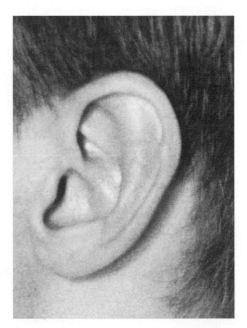

FIGURE 3-8.   Small Earlobes.   The subject in this photograph has a small earlobe, which shows that he focuses on the present and hasn't yet started planning for the future.

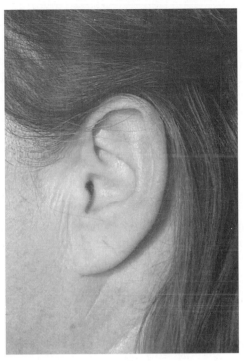

FIGURE 3-9.   **Attached Earlobes.** This photograph illustrates an attached earlobe and a person who is attached to her family.

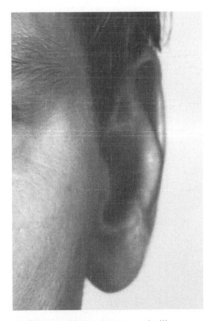

FIGURE 3-10.   **Detached Earlobes.** This photograph illustrates a detached earlobe and a person who creates friendships that become like family.

Most people have earlobes that are partially attached, which is considered healthy. They are close to some members of their birth family or family of origin but are also capable of creating a spiritual family of like-minded friends.

Placement of the ears also tells a tale. Measure the height of the ears in relationship to the rest of the face. From the side, draw a line from the top of the ear to the front of the face; the line will come across to either the forehead, the eyebrows, the eyes, or somewhere on the nose. Generally, the higher the ears, the younger that person "comes into his or her own." These people figure out what they want to do with their lives sooner. High ears are also a sign of a person who started working very young. This was traditionally seen as a sign of fame, because the younger you start working in your chosen profession, the more likely you are to become well known in your field. Many world-famous people have very high ears.

Ears that measure across to the forehead (Figure 3-11) indicate a person who is already on path by their twenties. If they measure across to the eyebrows, the person is on path by the early thirties. When the measure hits the eyes, is the person is on path by the late thirties (Figure 3-12), and a measure that reaches the nose indicates finding the path in the forties. Ears that are very low are considered a sign of a person with some possible mental deficiencies. However, it must be noted that Ronald Reagan had very low ears and did achieve fame. Although he was an actor when young, his roles were mostly forgettable. His true fame came very late in life when he entered politics: He was the consummate late bloomer.

Ears that are set close to the head (Figure 3-13) indicate a good listener and someone who has good hearing ability. An individual with ears that protrude from

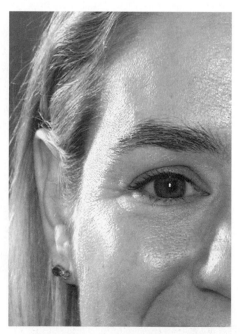

FIGURE 3-11.   High Ears.   The subject in this photograph has a high ear, which means she will come in to her own around her early 30s—her ear is as high as her eyebrow.

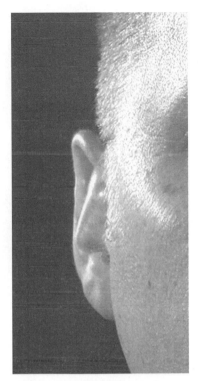

FIGURE 3-12.   **Low Ears.**   The subject in this photograph has a lower ear, which shows he will come into his own in his mid- to late 30s—his ear lines up with his eyes.

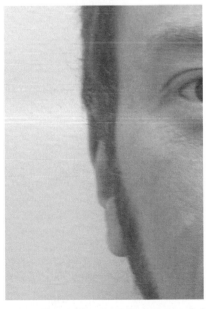

FIGURE 3-13.   **Close-set Ears.**   The subject in this photograph has an ear set very close to his head. He is a good listener and may have the ability to hear more than one conversation at a time.

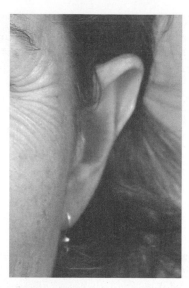

FIGURE 3-14.   Ears Set off the Face.   The subject in this photograph has an ear that is set off the face. This shows that she is stubborn about following directions and sometimes hears only what she wants to hear.

the head (Figure 3-14) doesn't like to listen to advice. This trait is called *auditory stubbornness.* The ancient Chinese said people with this trait "only hear what they want to hear."

HAIRLINE

The hairline is considered a minor water area and mainly represents the effects of fear in childhood and adolescence. In ancient Chinese face reading, this area was called "mother's influence." The saying was, "Your mother will always be your mother, even when you grow up." This meant individuals with a hairline that shows this influence are heavily impressed by the teachings of their mothers and keep them internalized; they end up living by these teachings even when they are away from their mothers. This is a belief system that is very hard to shake. The influence isn't always from the mother, however. It could be from any person who takes on the role of socializing a child. This could be a father, a grandparent, a nanny, or a teacher. They teach a child to conform to society's rules. These rules were and are taught by fear: Parents scare their children into looking before they cross the street, or they teach manners by threatening them with eventual censure from others.

The most socialized person will have a strong mother's influence. Mother's influence is shown by the lowering of the hairline on the sides of the forehead to create an oval or triangular look, as shown in Figure 3-15. Often many little flyaway hairs reside here. The closer the hairline is to the eyebrows, the more repressive the childhood.

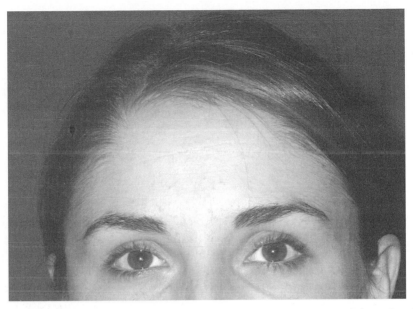

FIGURE 3-15.   Mother's Influence Hairline.   The subject in this photograph has a lovely oval forehead with characteristic small ears on the side. This means that she was heavily influenced by her mother's teachings and most likely has excellent social skills and manners.

People who were heavily socialized may need to be liberated from some of their beliefs, but they usually have excellent manners and are very polite. Such a person has been heavily trained and usually is concerned about other people's opinions and feelings. They know how to behave in high society, even if they haven't come from there.

One of my clients appeared to have very proper manners when she came in. When I questioned her about the very heavy mother's influence she showed, she assured me that she had learned no manners from her mother at all. In fact, she came from what she considered a very low-class family. Her family upset her so much that she used to sit in front of the fancy dress store in her small Texas town and watch all of the beautiful and rich women go in. She was so impressed by them that she decided to figure out how to be like them. She watched them for years and read every book on etiquette and fashion she could find. When she was old enough, she got a job in that store and went home and sewed dresses like the ones she couldn't afford so that she could look like the women she had watched. She watched and learned and listened. She changed the patterns of her speech and the way she walked. She modeled herself after the women she admired and ended up socializing herself!

The higher or broader the forehead, the freer the childhood was from rules, or the less a person paid attention to the socialization that was taught. A person with a more open forehead does not necessarily lack manners. Rather, an open forehead indicates a lack of concern about rules or the effects of breaking them. These people are more willing to risk censure or are less concerned about other people's opinions. A hairline that is squared or angular in the corners (Figure 3-16) indicates a person who likes to experiment with life despite the consequences of the experimentation. Such an individual is more rebellious about the rules and less impacted by disapproval.

A hairline that recedes in the corners on the diagonal (Figure 3-17) is not just a sign of losing hair. This type of hairline indicates an expansive thinker and someone who thinks "outside the box." People with this trait have an extrapolative mind that jumps to conclusions or answers before all of the information has been presented. It reminds me of cartoons in which a light bulb goes off in a person's head, and there is an *Aha!* This kind of thinking is often intuitive and progressive.

Balding or the lack of an obvious upper hairline is considered a positive attribute in Chinese face reading. My father was bald, and one of his favorite sayings that my mom told him was, "You will never see a bald beggar." The ancient Chinese believed bald men had more drive for both work and sex and would always end up successful. You would never see them begging because they liked to work. My father was very proud of being bald because of this.

The widow's peak, as shown in Figure 3-18, is another curious trait of the hairline. A widow's peak occurs when the hair comes down to a point in the middle of the forehead. It is considered a very magnetic and attractive feature. Studies have shown people prefer politicians who have this trait. It is a subliminal universal attractant.

In Chinese face reading, a woman with a widow's peak possesses a large quantity of primal water energy. This seductive quality is an outward expression of deep female power. Nothing has to be done to express this power; it is embodied and can be turned on or off. Great screen actresses have mastered this ability. Marilyn

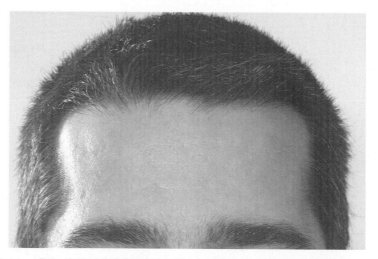

FIGURE 3-16. Experimental Forehead. The subject in this photograph has a broad hairline, which indicates the desire to experiment with his life and possibly rebel against conformity.

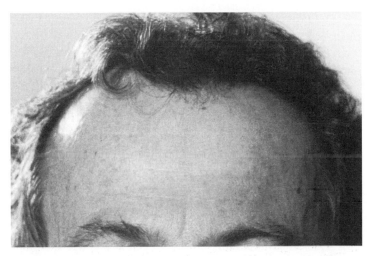

FIGURE 3-17.   Extrapolative Forehead.   The subject in this photograph has a forehead that goes back strongly in the corners and shows a mind that finds answers to difficult problems in an intuitive way.

Monroe, for example, was known to be able to walk down the street unnoticed until she decided to become "Marilyn" and turned on her seductiveness. Men were known to turn suddenly and stare as they felt the waves of her female power hit them.

The ancient Chinese believed women with widow's peaks easily attract boyfriends or husbands. This may explain the term's origin: These women don't stay widows for long, unless they want to. When one mate is on the way out, another one is usually waiting or shows up very soon after.

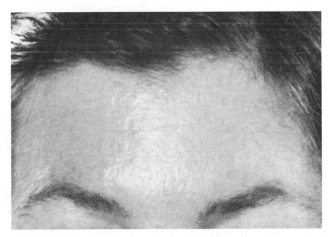

FIGURE 3-18.   Widow's Peak.   In this photograph, you can see the widow's peak that helps this woman attract the opposite sex easily.

This is a trait that can be cultivated. I once had a class of 14 women, five of whom had widow's peaks, and all five were involved in relationships. The other nine wanted to know how to find a mate as well. So we performed an experiment. I had every woman without a widow's peak practice feeling seductive. I had them imagine walking into a party where everyone was going to admire them. I had them do anything that made them feel more feminine—go buy some new clothes, get a new hairstyle, try a new lipstick color. I cautioned them not to turn this trait off when men approached. It turned out all the women knew how to do it but were afraid of getting too much attention. When they turned it off, they felt safer, yet they felt unattractive because no one ever approached them.

By the end of 10 weeks, every woman had started growing a widow's peak! I had one student who had men flying in from Chicago to take her to lunch. One woman got engaged, and another had more dates in those weeks than she had had in 5 years. Most of them ended up in a relationship. One of the students told me her new boyfriend had wanted to ask her out for almost a year, but she had never seemed available until one day he got the signal!

Men have a variation of this trait as well. The M-shaped hairline (Figure 3-19) is also attractive but has less to do with seduction. In men, this is a trait of enhanced creativity and sensitivity. These are the men who aren't afraid of having deep feelings and being expressive. They are the artist types. This is a special kind of attraction that draws people to these men.

UPPER FOREHEAD

The next area that relates to the water element is the upper forehead. This area is called "inheritance"; people with a rounded protrusion here on either one or both

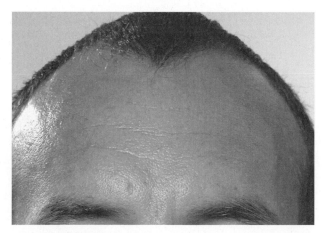

FIGURE 3-19.   M-shaped Hairline.   In this photograph, you can see the M-shaped hairline, which indicates that this man has a great deal of creativity and sensitivity.

sides have inherited talents and abilities from their ancestors. This area indicates the strength of the genetic gifts that have been given before birth. It may also indicate a literal inheritance that will be received after family members pass away, from artifacts to money.

A protruding right side of the upper forehead indicates inheritance primarily from the mother's family, whereas a left-sided dominance indicates the father's family has more influence. A completely rounded upper forehead indicates that the inheritance on both sides has similarities and is therefore amplified. For example, I come from two families that are from entirely different parts of the world and are of different races, yet both sides have members who are serious scholars, professors, musicians, and cooks. Therefore, in me, these traits are doubled. No wonder I am a college professor, an avid reader and researcher, and a singer and I have an overwhelming passion for cooking. It's in my DNA!

A rounded forehead (Figure 3-20) is also considered a sign of an imaginative mind, and the traits that fuel this kind of thinking are no doubt inherited. A dip in the center of the forehead or a separation of the two sides indicate a person whose ancestry on both sides is very different and may even be diametrically opposed. Balancing these opposing traits is quite challenging, and most people spend their entire lives trying to do so.

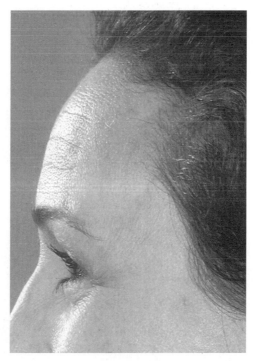

FIGURE 3-20.   **Rounded Forehead.**   This rounded forehead, viewed from the side, shows this woman's imaginative mind.

A flatter forehead (Figure 3-21) indicates a person who is a linear thinker and is less involved with ancestral talents and abilities. These individuals need to make their own way in the world willingly and are less bound by their inheritance. A forehead that slants back (Figure 3-22) indicates a person who is good at making deals and negotiating.

A high forehead (Figure 3-23) indicates a philosophical and intellectual mind. A person with this trait learns easily from books, school, and other people. A low forehead (Figure 3-24) indicates a person who learns best from experience, which is sometimes the best teacher.

UNDER-EYE AREA

The under-eye area is the best area on the face for evaluating the physical functioning of the kidneys. If the skin under the eye sinks down significantly deeper than the skin of the cheekbone, the individual has a condition of water deficiency or dehydration. When this area is also dark, the condition is considered

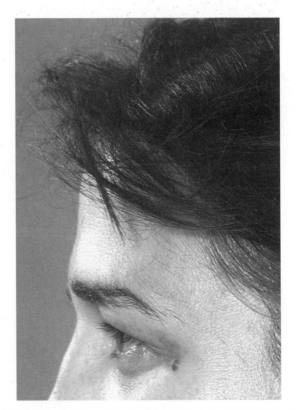

FIGURE 3-21.   **Straight Forehead.**   This straight forehead, viewed from the side, shows this woman's linear mind.

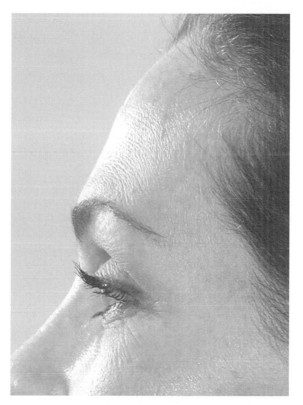

FIGURE 3-22. **Slanted Forehead.** This slanted forehead, viewed from the side, shows this woman's facile mind and negotiating ability.

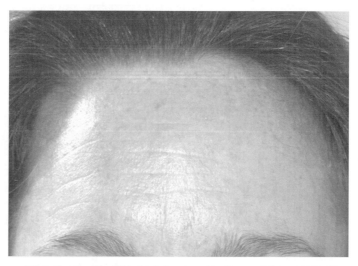

FIGURE 3-23. **High Forehead.** This high forehead indicates this man's intellectual mind and philosophical nature.

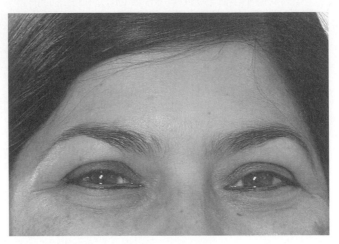

FIGURE 3-24.   **Low Forehead.** This low forehead indicates this woman's need to learn things from experience.

chronic. It could be a sign of allergies, exhaustion, or a psychological condition called *unshed tears from the past.* An under-eye area that is puffy and has "bags" shows kidney stagnation. This may be caused by excess mineralization of the body or tears ready to be shed from a recent hurt. This area is discussed in depth in Chapter 9.

PHILTRUM

The philtrum is the groove between the nose and mouth. This area was originally called "fertility and creativity" and was considered the lifeline of the face. Longevity is predicted by how long or wide or deep it was. If it is wider across the top, your best health was in childhood. If it is wider across the middle, midlife is your healthiest time. If it is wider across the bottom, old age is destined to be a healthy period (Figure 3-25). If this groove is straight and parallel and deep (Figure 3-26), your entire life is considered balanced in terms of health. If the groove is very narrow, even if long, your health is considered precarious throughout life.

This area also corresponds to the reproductive area of the body and shows how well it functions. Traditionally, it was believed that if you had a strong groove, you had the ability and energy to have and raise a large number of children. This ensured you would be taken care of in old age and therefore would live longer. You could expect to be revered in your old age as the head of your family and finally achieve the recognition you deserved. Any extraneous markings on the groove indicates a problem with fertility. A small philtrum (Figure 3-27) indicates fewer potential children and decreased fertility.

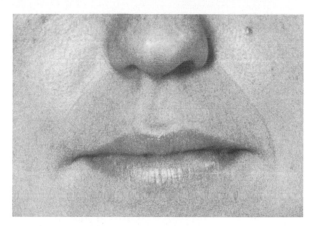

FIGURE 3-25.   **Wide, Deep Philtrum.**   The wide, deep philtrum pictured here is indicative of great creativity and fertility and shows potential good health in this woman's old age.

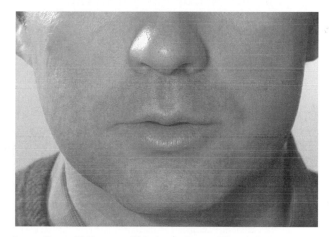

FIGURE 3-26.   **Long, Deep Philtrum.**   This long, deep philtrum is indicative of good creativity and fertility, especially in youth, and fairly consistent good health throughout this man's life.

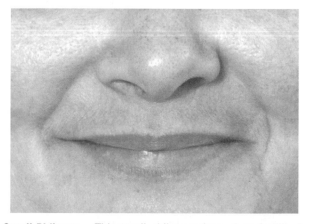

FIGURE 3-27.   **Small Philtrum.**   This small philtrum shows less fertility because it is not a very long or wide groove, but its depth shows she is a creative woman.

If you had a strong philtrum, yet did not have any children, you were advised to become extremely creative or you would not live as long. Creativity gives more meaning to life and gives a person a reason to live longer.

The more esoteric meaning of this area was "immortality." The stronger the groove, the more capable you were of becoming immortal. Immortality was an obsession for the Chinese, and they searched far and wide for magic elixirs that would let them live forever. Ultimately, they determined that there were only a few ways to become immortal. The first was the traditional route of having offspring who would carry on your genes, your talents, and your teachings. This was "carrying on the family name," and each generation was instructed to make this name a prouder one than it already was.

Another way to become immortal was to become a scholar, an artist, or a philosopher. These were considered noble professions that were honored by the government. You were expected to cultivate your talents and knowledge. After a lifetime of work, you were able to leave a legacy of your study through writings or teachings or to show your talent through your artistic endeavors.

The last way to become immortal was to become enlightened. This was the hardest path because you had to leave everything behind. You had to eliminate attachment to all material things, cultivate the truths of the universe, and live according to them. Eventually, you would transcend the body to become spirit and be revered forever.

The correlation of immortality to the kidneys is an interesting one. Because the *jing* determines a person's potential life span, this is one of the areas that shows how capable a person is of transcending the limits of the human body to live beyond the time allotted in physical form. Without creativity, life becomes mundane. With a strong desire to create, people have to find outlets that allow their creativity to flourish.

THE CHIN

The chin is an indicator of the emotional strength of the kidneys. This is a feature that can be grown, although bone development takes some time to accomplish. Generally speaking, the stronger the chin, the stronger the will. This is especially true when the chin is long. Will can be a good trait or a bad trait, depending on perspective. Willfulness can be dangerous. From experience I have learned that pushing the square peg into the round hole is not usually a wise thing to do. However, being willing is usually an advantageous thing. The long chin (Figure 3-28) is also considered a sign of longevity because it involves the will to live and a person who will probably work long into old age. A small chin (Figure 3-29) is a sign of less will but also a gentler and more easy-going personality. A person with a small chin is advised to retire early to enjoy the last part of life without effort. A turned-up chin (Figure 3-30) is a sign of stubbornness.

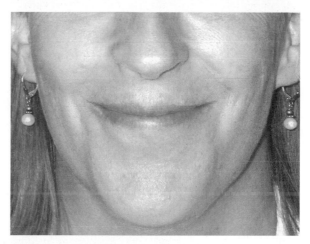

FIGURE 3-28. **Strong Chin.** The subject in this photo has a very strong and long chin, which are both signs of a very strong will.

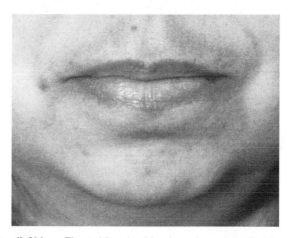

FIGURE 3-29. **Small Chin.** The subject in this photo has a small chin, which indicates the desire to retire early and an easygoing nature.

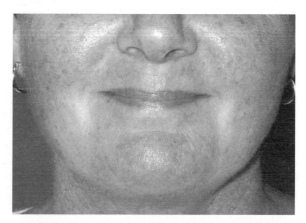

FIGURE 3-30. **Turned-up Chin.** The turned-up chin in this photo indicates this woman's stubborn streak. She digs her heels in when necessary and won't budge.

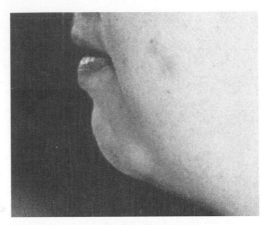

FIGURE 3-31.   Receding Chin.   The receding chin in this photo indicates that this woman has been dominated in the past but is most likely a champion of the underdog now.

A receding chin (Figure 3-31) indicates a curious mixture of traits. Traditionally, this has been viewed as a weak chin. However, individuals with receding chins have actually been dominated by someone else's will and were not allowed to develop their own. This does not mean that the person is easily dominated now. In fact, most people with receding chins are quite resistant to being dominated and actively fight against it. These people are most often champions of the underdog because they have been one and are actively seeking to become more willful.

The shape of the chin also has meaning. Square chins (Figure 3-32) show emotional strength and practicality. Rounded chins (Figure 3-33) show diplomacy and an even disposition. Pointed chins (Figure 3-34) show indecisiveness and emotionality.

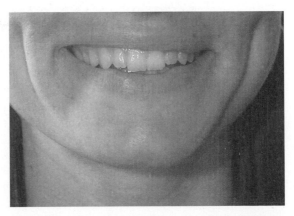

FIGURE 3-32.   Square Chin.   The squared chin in this photo belongs to a woman who is emotionally strong and is practical about the expression of her emotions.

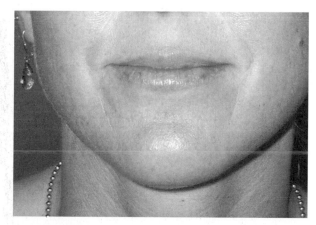

FIGURE 3-33.   Rounded Chin.   The rounded chin in this photo belongs to a woman who is diplomatic and even-tempered.

Stubbornness is a trait best seen from the side and is relatively deceptive. The chin looks pushed up and in. The more strongly the chin tilts up or the more it is pushed in, the more tenacious and resistant the individual is to moving. People with this kind of chin are not considered flexible or easygoing. They are pugnacious and resistant to change. When combined with a strong jaw, they are almost immovable. But that leads us into the wood element features.

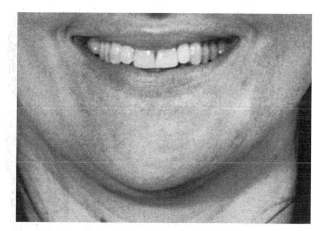

FIGURE 3-34.   Pointed Chin.   The pointed chin in this photo belongs to a woman who is emotional, yet indecisive.

4 / *The Wood Features and Traits*

"Wood is as forceful and determined as the wind, as supple as a spreading aspen stretching into a bright cloudless sky."
HARRIET BIENFIELD AND EFREM KORNGOLD, *BETWEEN HEAVEN AND EARTH*[1]

The strength of wood is shown in the power of the features that correspond to the liver. The liver is an amazing organ. It enjoys processing toxins and then regenerating. It relishes in dealing with poisonous substances and clearing them from the body, unless, of course, it has to deal with too many. This physical trait is also manifested emotionally. People with strong wood have the ability to get very angry and enjoy expressing themselves through their tempers. This can manifest as work, athleticism, and a fighting spirit. Although anger can be toxic, it is dangerous to wood people only when used too much or too little. Wood people feel alive when in action, and their anger is a wonderfully motivating force for them. Because the liver also handles environmental toxins, people with strong liver *qi* can process drugs and alcohol better and react very well to herbal medicines, which are part of the wood family in nature but are also mildly toxic. In fact, only people with strong liver *qi* are capable of substance abuse, although this does not mean they will abuse substances. Most alcoholics have very strong eyebrows. People with limited liver *qi* would suffer from alcohol poisoning long before they became alcoholics.

The true strength of the wood element is shown in the ability to be active, both physically and emotionally. The features associated with the liver show an orientation toward action, temper, the desire for altered states, determination, and issues with authority. The vital feature of the wood element is the eyebrows, and this is the feature most closely associated with the functioning of the liver.

---

[1]Bienfield H, Korngold E: *Between Heaven and Earth*, New York, Ballantine Books, 1991.

EYEBROWS

There are many shapes and sizes of eyebrows, but the most important quality about them is their size. Eyebrow hairs are called "leaves of the tree" and symbolize the primal strength of the growing tree. Large, long, bushy, wiry, or thick eyebrows show tremendous liver *qi* and the ability to express anger, drive, and passion (Figures 4-1 and 4-2). This is comparable to a tree with a big trunk and many strong leaves or needles. People with thick or big eyebrows are showing that they are rigid

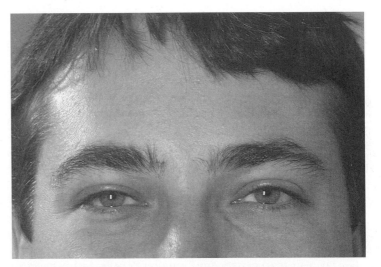

FIGURE 4-1. The subject in this photo has strong eyebrows, which indicates that he also has a strong liver and a temper to match.

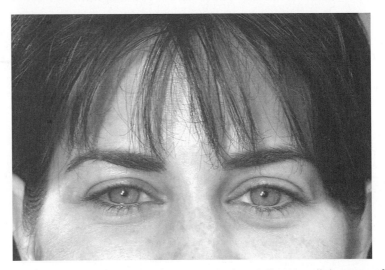

FIGURE 4-2. The subject in this photo has strong eyebrows that are a little more refined than those in Figure 4-1. She also has a strong liver and a big temper but can repress it more easily.

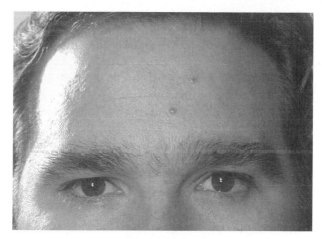

FIGURE 4-3.   The subject in this photo has thick eyebrows, which shows a powerful liver and a strong drive.

in their thinking and have reactive natures. People with thick or big eyebrows (Figure 4-3) see threats in many actions or words that other people would overlook. They are antagonized easily. Eyebrows with fine, soft, or short hairs (Figure 4-4) are much more like delicate trees that sway in the wind with fluttering leaves. Individuals with these eyebrows tend to go with the flow more and can't be bothered to spend much time upset. Their liver *qi* may not be as powerful, but the flexibility of these individuals is an asset in life.

The thicker the eyebrows are, the more assertive someone is. When there is additional bushiness or coarseness of hair, you have a person who won't take no for

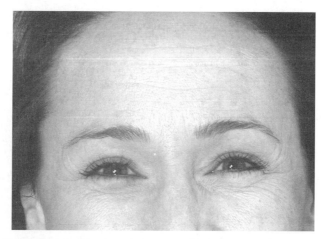

FIGURE 4-4.   The subject in this photo has very refined eyebrows, which is an indication of a more passive temperament. Although she undoubtedly gets angry on occasion, anger is not a comfortable emotion for her.

an answer. Such individuals could be referred to as pushy, even domineering. They are capable of volcanic anger but also great humanitarianism, although a strong wood person helps by leading the horses to water and then pushing their heads in to make them drink!

Eyebrows that grow together above the nose, a "unibrow" (Figure 4-5), are a sign of extra aggression. Unfortunately, it is also a sign that other people interpret as threatening. They then pick fights with these unibrowed people because they are so intimidated by their power. In actuality, people with a unibrow work very hard to control their explosive temper and aggressive nature and allow this powerful energy to emerge only on the playing field. In its most positive light, the unibrow is an extremely useful trait for contact sports. People with very strong eyebrows or a unibrow are most likely to hold or control their tempers because they know just how big their anger can be. Even they are afraid of that release. They tend to simmer and stew if they don't have an outlet, which can lead to depression. Therefore they need to participate in physical activity to work the tension and anger out of their body.

On the other hand, people with thin or soft eyebrows are easy-going and much more passive. They are perceived as kind and gentle, but in reality they have a shorter fuse on their temper when they are overloaded. They can be high-strung and volatile; they snap instead of explode and get over it very quickly. They get exhausted by arguments, rarely feel better after they have gotten things off their chest, and prefer everyone to just get along. They try to cultivate peace and harmony and have a very poor tolerance of alcohol and drugs. However, they can adapt readily to changing situations without getting rattled.

One of the ways to discover hidden liver qi is to rub the eyebrows backward. Even if the eyebrows appear to be very shapely and smooth or have been managed by tweezing, the true test is to check the eyebrow hair for tensile strength (Figure 4-6).

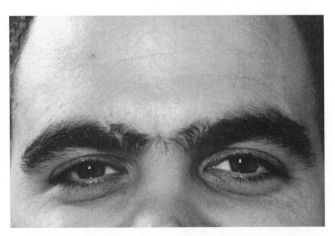

FIGURE 4-5.   The subject in this photo has eyebrow hairs between his eyebrows, which is a sign of aggressiveness and an explosive temper. This trait would be especially useful in sports.

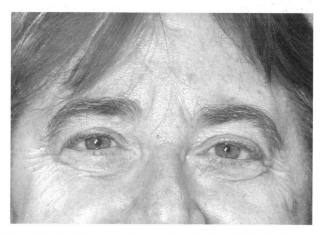

FIGURE 4-6.   The subject in this photo has eyebrow hairs with body. They would be resistant to being pushed, and so is she.

If the hair does not bend back easily, you have a person with automatic resistance and hidden liver qi. While they may outwardly appear to be cooperative and accommodating, they are not that easy-going.

Eyebrow hairs that grow long and wild are called "mad scientist's eyebrows" (Figure 4-7). These eyebrow hairs look like they have a mind of their own and belong to owners that definitely have unusual minds. This trait is especially potent when seen on a person under the age of 60. People with this trait think out of the box. They are primarily men and are known as "Mr. Fix-its." They like nothing more than to have a problem to solve, and live for the time when the light bulb goes off in their heads and they come up with a brilliant solution. The only problem with

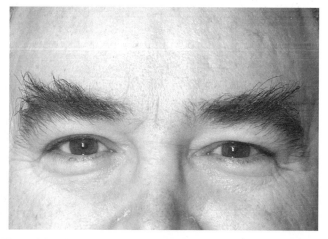

FIGURE 4-7.   The subject in this photo has eyebrow hairs that grow very long and wild. This indicates an inventive mind and a Mr. Fixit personality.

these occasionally inspired thinkers is that they sometimes forget that not all of their ideas are brilliant. They can get lost in their pondering and not listen or pay attention to what is going on around them. They have a keen ability to focus when necessary for the pure pleasure of being right and making things work. This is a highly valuable trait found in inventors.

As the hairs of the eyebrows are leaves of the tree, the length of the eyebrow shows how long the branch is (Figure 4-8). The longer the branch, the more leaves it can grow. Leaves are comparable to friends. Traditionally, the longer the eyebrows, the more friends a person is capable of having. This is because people with the wood element can be the most humanitarian when they use their liver qi in mature and spiritual ways. Unfortunately, when they have not evolved spiritually they can be very judgmental and determined to make people change. People with lots of eyebrow hairs have the energy to have lots of friends and surround themselves with people who appreciate their wood temperament. Wood people make good friends.

Shorter eyebrows (Figure 4-9) belong to people who are very independent. They insist on doing everything they possibly can by themselves. They don't have as many friends because they don't have the extra energy to take care of a lot of relationships. They usually manage their energy carefully and can only afford to have few very close friends whom they can trust and who don't demand too much of them. They don't ask for help and don't want to receive any because it would make them beholden to others. These short eyebrows are correlated to the gallbladder, which is the scorekeeper of the body. People with short eyebrows have a minor deficiency in the gallbladder and can't handle too much fat in their diet or too many favors from their friends. Because they keep tabs, they can't rest until they have repaid the favor, usually doubling the amount or effort. This leaves them exhausted and thus limits the number of people they can "owe." Also, if they keep giving and never getting back, the gallbladder goes into resentment mode, which weakens it even more.

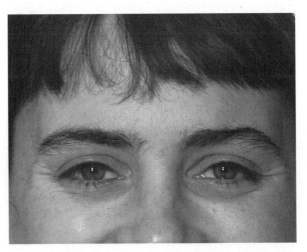

FIGURE 4-8.   The subject in this photo has very long eyebrows and shows the ability to have a lot of friends.

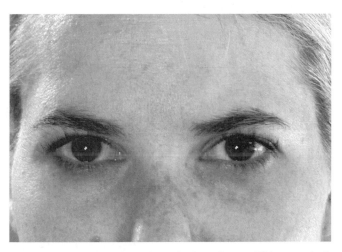

FIGURE 4-9.   The subject in this photo has short eyebrows. This reveals her independent personality and her desire to do things for herself.

The downside of short eyebrows is that these people can end up feeling lonely and unloved. They genuinely like people but avoid getting too involved with very many. Because they never ask for help, people assume that they have everything under control and are perfectly self-sufficient. Other people are not used to having them need anything, so they don't notice the hints that these subtle people emit when they are in need. Because they hint instead of ask, they rely on close friends and family members to read the signs and offer help.

The next trait to examine is the arch of the eyebrow. The shape of the arch determines the action orientation of a person (Figure 4-10). The stronger the arch,

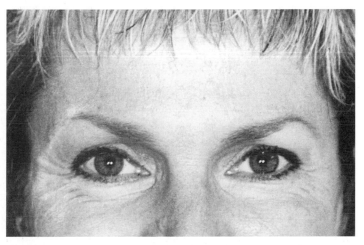

FIGURE 4-10.   The subject in this photo has eyebrows that go straight up. When she wants to get something done, she just does it. You don't have to wait on her at all.

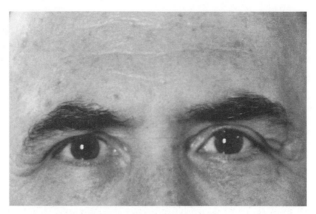

FIGURE 4-11.   The subject in this photo has eyebrows with a strong arch. He moves fast and likes to get things done quickly.

the more active or decisive the person will be. Eyebrows that slant directly upward from the inside corner like a straight line belong to people who act fast. Very reminiscent of the Nike motto, "Just do it!" these people like to do and do it now. They don't wait for all the information because they don't like waiting around. These individuals have a strong streak of impatience. They think on their feet and decide quickly, so they are sometimes seen as rash and impetuous.

Eyebrows that are arched in the middle so that each eyebrow looks like an upside-down **V**, belong to people who work their way into decisiveness but are still quick to act (Figure 4-11). They need to think about things just a little bit, but once they decide, they go for it. Then they move quickly and forcefully. There is an aggressive quality to their action.

Straight eyebrows (Figure 4-12) reveal a person who likes to mull over decisions and takes time deciding. These kinds of people act eventually but after much

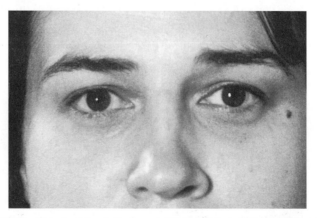

FIGURE 4-12.   The subject in this photo has eyebrows that are fairly straight. She does things at her own, consistent pace.

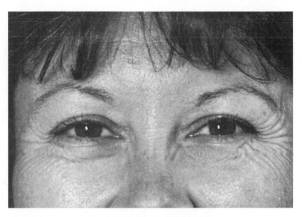

FIGURE 4-13.   The subject in this photo has eyebrows that naturally curve. She possesses feminine wiles and knows how to work with people, especially men.

deliberation and are slower to react overall. They are much more likely to go along with someone else's ideas or plans and are a good match for people with strongly arched or v-shaped eyebrows.

Eyebrows that are very rounded and curved over the eye (Figure 4-13) are called the "concubine's eyebrows." These eyebrows are often deliberately shaped this way by women who tweeze their eyebrows but are most powerful when natural. It is also an eyebrow shape that is sometimes drawn in with an eyebrow pencil after severe tweezing or shaving of the natural brow. These eyebrows belong to women who have feminine wiles. Instead of using their temper, they use their charm to cajole and tempt others to get their needs met. This is considered primarily a female trait.

BROW BONES

Brow bones are much more common in men than in women. The development of the ridge of bone over the eyebrow correlates to higher doses of testosterone, which the liver is responsible for circulating, and these ridges are considered a sign of masculinity. Women do have them, but they are usually stronger in men. There are several different degrees of protrusion. In general, the stronger the brow bone, the more dominance this person desires or asserts (Figure 4-14). Brow bones signify an automatic resistance to authority and being told what to do. These ridges are signs of power and leadership ability. They are often associated with rigid and dogmatic thinking. You can be assured that these people have a tremendous physical presence. They are usually very athletic and tough. They absolutely hate being told what to do and barely tolerate having someone else in charge. They are much happier when they are in charge and on top. They need to be dominant in their personal relationships and are authoritarian parents whose motto is "my way is the only way."

If there is a dip in the middle of the brow ridge, you have a person who is a lot easier to manage. These people also hate being told what to do but seem to take

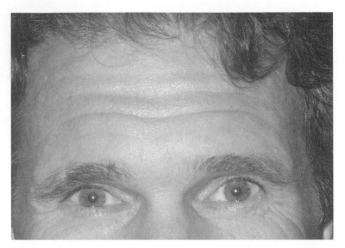

FIGURE 4-14.   The subject in this photo has very strong brow bones. This indicates that he doesn't like being told what to do and would much prefer to be the one doing the telling.

it a lot better when they are asked nicely. For them, how they are asked is more important than what they are asked to do. They still want to be in charge but are happy with the appearance or even the illusion of power. They bristle at orders unless they respect their superior. They have little tolerance for bosses who are weak or ineffective when they know they could do a better job because their browbone is not quite as pronounced and they are usually more flexible. Although they still have issues with authority, they handle overseeing others better and could be considered authoritative instead of authoritarian.

THE SEAT OF THE STAMP

In ancient China, everyone who was intelligent, talented, or politically savvy was given a position in the hierarchical government. To signify position, each person was given a personalized chop, a signature stamp of varying size, to sign correspondence or work. The higher the position a person held, the bigger the chop. This was a sign of their power.

On the face, there is an equivalent sign for potential power. The area between the eyebrows above the nose is called the "seat of the stamp" or the "father's influence" area. This area is a minor liver area that corresponds to a person's issues with anger (from the past) that have to do with discipline, usually involving the father or the person who took the *yang* parental role. If this area is broad and clear, and the eyebrows are spaced far apart, it means that this person had a benevolent father figure. The breadth of this area indicates a father's blessing, like having a father or mentor who encouraged business success and taught about the natural order of things (Figure 4-15). These people have the patience to wait their turn to rise up the ladder. They seldom burn bridges and usually

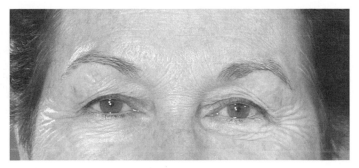

FIGURE 4-15. The width between this woman's eyebrows shows a good relationship with her father or other dominant role model. This also means that she does not have issues with authority.

gain a reputation of being easy to get along with. There is also an ability to assess the right time to make a move to ensure their promotion.

When the eyebrows are close together and the area between the brows is narrow, you have a person with impatience to succeed (Figure 4-16). They don't want to wait their turn to move up in the hierarchy. They usually have some issues with discipline from the past and believe they are deserving of promotion because they are smarter, harder working, or otherwise more qualified than those above them. This is especially true if the eyebrows are held closer together with a frown. These people are lone wolves and like to work independently. They prefer to be in business for themselves, where they are the boss. In organizations, they do best in situations where they are not heavily supervised. They rebel when given negative reviews and are touchy about criticism or perceived slights. They get irritated when their superiors act (in their opinion) incompetently. Although these kinds of people commonly work in corporations, they are usually considered slightly rebellious or powerful proponents of change.

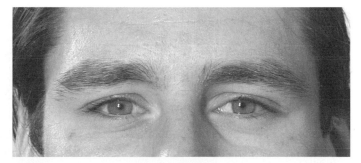

FIGURE 4-16. The narrowness between this man's eyebrows indicates that he has issues with anger and has trouble working within a hierarchy. He may be happiest going into business for himself or getting a job where he is given a lot of freedom.

If the area between the eyebrows is marked by lines, an individual is impatient, irritable, or easily annoyed or frustrated. The liver is either overloaded with old anger or tired and incapable of handling any new anger. In either case, this area shows a kind of reactivity that is quick to respond to any form of attack from outside. For example, a person who squints a lot in bright sunshine will get these lines, but you have to ask why they don't wear sunglasses. They obviously enjoy being aggravated by the sun, and they will also have the tendency to be irritable in response to any other form of attack, even a provocative question. The bigger, deeper, or stronger the line, the older the issues are, or the more tired the liver is from past or current anger or overwork.

The strongest line is called the "suspended sword." It is a single line between the eyebrows that is very deep (Figure 4-17). It is a symbol that the liver is cut in half and that at some point, the issues behind this marking will stop forward progress because the sword will drop and cut off the foot. This sign is also called "estrangement." It is considered a sign of estrangement from father, estrangement from sons, or estrangement from the person's own male or yang energy. It is correlated with a person using only half of the liver *qi*. This condition usually arises when a person has had a father (or dominant parent) who had a lot of rage. Consequently, these children grow up believing that anger is very dangerous and destructive, and they then suppress their own anger, which bottles up the liver *qi*. They may have rage that they do not express because they are so afraid of it and have seen the damage it can cause or they grew up in a family in which anger was not allowed. In either case, they are not accessing their full power. If they work through their issues about anger and learn how to use it appropriately, they discover that they have tremendous energy reserves that are untapped.

I once had a client, Bob, who had a line so deep that it looked like a canyon on his forehead. Bob had some serious estrangement issues. His father had been an angry alcoholic and was dead. His son was an angry alcoholic and wouldn't talk to him any more. Bob never drank because he was so afraid of becoming an alcoholic like his father or his son. He avoided getting angry because he was terrified that he

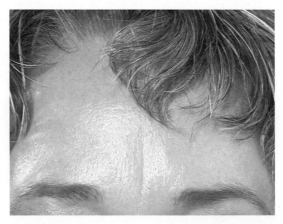

FIGURE 4-17. Although this is a very small suspended sword or line between her eyebrows, it does show that she is using only half of her liver *qi* and power.

would kill someone if he let it out. His father had beaten him badly, and he knew that he too was capable of this kind of rage. In looking at this marking, I realized that he had suppressed so much of his powerful liver *qi* that he had held himself back from business success. People always took advantage of him, and he would fume internally but never express it. Consequently, he had high blood pressure, heart disease, and a chronically enlarged liver. I counseled him for quite a while about what he could do to work through his issues and gave him referrals to a variety of therapists. To my surprise, Bob did what I had never seen before. Six months later, the line was virtually gone.

In asking him what he had done, Bob told me that he reconciled with his son. He forgave his son for being like his father and realized that he also needed to forgive himself. He had taken much of the blame for his son's failure and believed that he had also been the cause of his father's anger. Bob was a deeply religious man and had prayed continuously, eventually surrendering his need to be in such strict control of himself. He also started an intense exercise program to work the old anger and tension out of his body. A therapist helped him see the past more clearly and from a new perspective. He stopped letting people take advantage of him so often and learned to say no without feeling guilt. It was really amazing how well he cleared his issues. In addition, his blood pressure dropped, his liver had returned to a more normal size, and his arrhythmia had lessened. He was on his way to better health by processing his issues with anger. The diminishing line on his face showed just how much work he had done. I was very proud of him, and, most important, his quality of life improved dramatically.

A single line that is smaller and fainter than the suspended sword is called the "suspended needle" (Figure 4-18). It is symbolic of smaller issues about anger that block forward progress because the needle will one day drop and stab the foot. This also impedes forward progress but is more of an annoyance than a hindrance. It shows estrangement primarily from the person's own male or yang side. These people are afraid to offend and, although they secretly believe that they should be

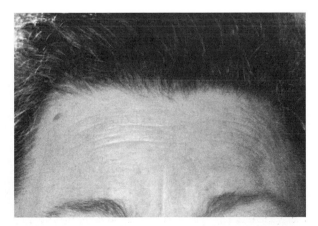

FIGURE 4-18. This very small line between her eyebrows indicates that this woman has repressed liver *qi* that she is not accessing for her growth and development.

given power, don't have the assertiveness to go for it. They instead get angry that they are passed over or left behind. This line signifies an inability to be as aggressive as is necessary for success. There is usually a dislike of other, more powerful people and a disdain for those who act aggressively. Individuals with this trait believe that they are assertive but are actually quite passive and prone to letting other people take advantage.

Two lines between the brows (Figure 4-19) indicate people who are impatient, irritable, easily annoyed, frustrated, or impatient. They either have lots of old anger that they don't want to let out all at once and so they spew it out in little bits, or they have a very tired liver that is overreactive to any supposed slight. The target of the irritation, frustration, or annoyance is rarely the one who caused it in the first place, so expressing it doesn't get rid of the old anger, a phenomenon called *displaced anger*. This is an extremely common marking in our stressful world because everyone seems to get annoyed or irritated with rush hour traffic, poor service, or other cranky people when they are really angry at someone or something else. This behavior has created an epidemic of lines between the brows in my clients and everywhere I look. People are lining up to get BoTox injections to paralyze the nerves in this area and get rid of these lines. It might be a lot smarter and a whole lot healthier to learn to express anger when needed and then let it go. We need to lighten up and get mad only at the things that are worth getting mad about.

Three or more lines (Figure 4-20) are actually a sign that the bearer had issues with anger in the past but has learned to manage the anger. These individuals can determine whether something is worth getting angry over or whether it is better to let it go. They have a more mature way of looking at anger and choose when and how to express it. They've done it all the different ways and have figured out what works for them.

The seat of the stamp area is also the opening to what is called the "third eye" and one of the most important *chakras*. The third eye is the ability to see beyond what is and see the deeper meaning. It is the ability to see through people and into universal truth. The ancient Chinese believed that the liver is the seat of the soul. They believed the liver has the ability to free the soul when it transcends the need to

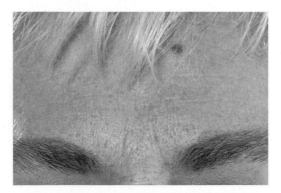

FIGURE 4-19. The subject in this photo has two lines between her eyebrows. These lines show that she often feels impatient, irritable, or annoyed.

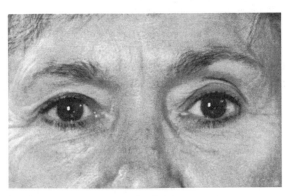

FIGURE 4-20.   The subject in this photo has three lines between her eyebrows. These lines indicate that although she has felt a lot of anger in the past, she now has a healthy relationship with this emotion. She has learned when to get angry, how much, and whether it is even worth expressing at all.

be angry. Anger and spirituality are mutually exclusive after a certain point in spiritual progress. To blame others, to hold grudges or resentment, and to hate are things that keep people in the past and hold the soul hostage. To free the soul and to open the third eye fully, people need to move into appreciation of all the things that got them where they are today. One of the steps to enlightenment is to find the reasons for everything that happened and to understand the importance of what happened. The realization that everything that has come before has led you to the place you are now is an evolved perspective and will get you where you want to go faster.

People who are on a spiritual path have indentations on the forehead of varying widths that show how "open" the third eye is (Figure 4-21). This is not a contest. It is only better to have an open third eye if you want to see. Some people are much happier living in denial, being justifiably angry, or believing what they are told. They don't need to have an open third eye. However, because the liver also determines drive, many people have the desire to explore or live in a quest mode and

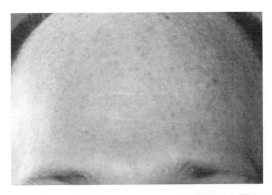

FIGURE 4-21.   The subject in this photo has a very open third eye. This allows him to see into situations and other people's motivations.

search for spiritual answers. These people have to let go of their socialization and their attachment to the collective belief systems with which they were raised. They will find teachers along their way. The markings of the third eye opening can have many shapes. Some of these shapes have particular meaning and are subject to interpretation.

A distinct line or ridge that forms a diagonal from the outer hairline down toward the outer eyebrow on the sides of the forehead reveals a person who has gone through some kind of spiritual awakening or has emerged from a period of deep darkness and has become more enlightened on the journey. This line is a sign of a very open third eye. It can be seen on people who have had near-death experiences, a huge "Aha" experience, or have gained wisdom from deep suffering. In any case, it is a sign of spiritual progress and knowledge gained the hard way.

TEMPLES

The temple area on either side of the forehead, past the eyes and before the hairline, indicates the "desire for altered states." It is a natural human desire to want to experience altered states, and the easiest way to do so is through alcohol or hallucinogenic substances. The desire for altered states has been observed in other animals as well. Elephants have been known to come from miles around to eat fermented fruit and get drunk, and birds love fermented berries. In the past, many cultures used these substances in religious ceremonies. They cultivated altered states as a way of achieving closeness to the spirit world. They wanted to have visions that would give their lives meaning. They were guided by a shaman or holy man in these visions; they were supervised while in these altered states and cared for when they came back to the present. These substances were not originally meant to be used recreationally, although they can be and have been abused throughout time.

The ideal state of this area is for the temples to be full and even plump. This kind of marking indicates people who live in the present. They usually do not have a strong desire to live in altered states and are happy with a simple life. They do not seek ecstatic states or experience the depths of despair. They just live.

However, there are a large number of people who actively seek altered states, and they represent a continuum of experiences. Those seeking altered states have indented temples, and they can be either dark or light. The bigger the indentation, the more these people seek altered states. It is most apparent in addicts or alcoholics and is very dark, but it is also just as apparent in yogis and other very spiritual people, whose temples are very light (Figure 4-22).

It is often easier to go to the dark side of the continuum. This includes all substance abuse, addictions, and some forms of mental illness. Individuals who choose these methods are self-medicating and often desperate to find answers to their problems. They make the initial choice to be self-destructive rather than constructive when faced with a problem, and this, when combined with a biochemical

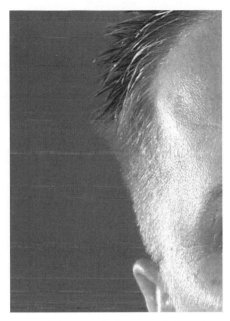

FIGURE 4-22. The subject in this photo has strong indentations in his forehead, but the coloration is very light. This indicates that he is either very spiritual or very creative and gets lost in a blissful state of being.

tendency toward depression or substance abuse, can lead to addiction or chronic self-destructive behavior.

The light side of altered states occurs when spiritual or creative activity produces a state of ecstasy and timelessness. It is achieved by cultivating the spiritual practice of mindlessness or by engaging in a pleasurable or creative activity that helps you transcend time and space. People in this state aren't aware of how long they are in it. Minutes seem like hours, and hours can seem like minutes. People often struggle to get to this state, but the reward is so great that they keep pursuing it. It is also very addictive. In actuality, it requires surrendering goals and is the effortless process of living fully and activating the unconscious. Mihaly Csikszentmihalyi first wrote about it from a scientific perspective in his book, *Flow: The Psychology of Optimal Experience.*[2] This kind of altered state shows up as a distinct indentation that is very light in coloration. People who master this form of altered states live in a more enlightened state of consciousness. They learn to transcend the laws of time and space.

I believe that the people who are most drawn to altered states are people seeking spirituality and creativity, but they are often misguided and fall into the trap of seeking escape from a painful reality or past instead of confronting it or

[2]Csikszentmihalyi M, *The Psychology of Optimal Experience*, New York, HarperCollins, 1991.

transcending it. They may suffer so deeply from the letdown after they have achieved flow that they fall into despair and have trouble getting up again. They need guides to steer them from dark to light. This is why many of the treatment options for alcohol and drug abuse emphasize spirituality, religion, and a higher power. It is an attempt to pull these people out of the dark side of altered states into the lighter side. It works—although slowly—because being light takes consistent effort and disciplined practice in surrendering the conscious self. The light side of altered states is worth achieving for those people who are willing to do the work, but it is really for those with an artist's soul or a spiritual calling. Otherwise, there is nothing wrong with living a worldly life. For many people, it is the preferred way of living.

EYE DEPTH

The depth of the eyes on the face shows whether someone is an introvert or an extrovert. You measure the depth of the eye by holding a pencil up vertically over your eye so that it touches both the browbone and cheekbone. Then, open and close your eye. If your eyelashes and eyelid do not hit the pencil, you have deep-set eyes. If your eyelashes and eyelid brush the pencil or almost get stuck, you have average-set eyes. If you cannot open your eyelid, you have protruding eyes.

Deep-set eyes belong to introverted people (Figure 4-23). These are deep thinkers and nontalkers. They live inside themselves most of the time. They have slower reaction times because they process information before acting on it. They watch other people before engaging in conversation and often have to be prompted to react. They need a lot of alone time and gain energy from recharging this way. If this area has a dark cast, it is a sign of depression.

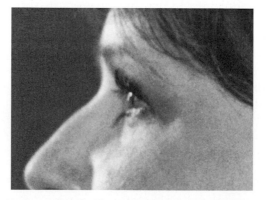

FIGURE 4-23. This woman has eyes that are set behind her brow bone. This is a sign of an introverted personality. She is probably shyer than she appears and also a quiet person.

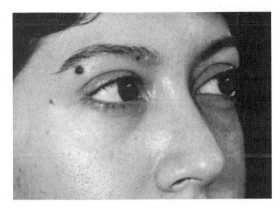

FIGURE 4-24.   The woman in this photo has eyes that are about equal to the protrusion of her brow bone. This is a sign of an extraverted personality and a sociable person.

Protruding eyes belong to bold and impulsive people. They speak or blurt out things before they think them through. They are quick to act and react. They are prone to thyroid problems because the liver overacts on the thyroid gland. They are social and they are recharged by being around other people. This is a problem for them because they dislike being alone. They think and process out loud and in the presence of others.

People with an average set to their eyes (Figure 4-24) are moderately sociable people who are moderate in their ability to act and react. They are primarily extraverted with some need for time alone.

SCLERA OF THE EYE

The sclera of the eye is the area of the face that most accurately shows the current physiological functioning of the liver. It comprises the whites of the eyes and is commonly known as a place that is connected to the liver because jaundice, which shows a diseased liver, creates yellow eye whites. Of course there are many other colors of sclera that are much less dangerous than that. Scleras are supposed to be white, white; scleras indicate a healthy liver. When the scleras are red, it is a sign of a tired liver. You have overused your liver *qi* and need to rest. When the eye whites are pale grayish/greenish/yellowish, you have a sign that the liver is slightly toxified. This is often a sign of an oncoming illness, such as the flu. In chronic disease, the scleras remain this color and darken with the severity of the illness.

JAW

The jaw is called the "roots of the tree." Strong roots or a big jaw (Figure 4-25) means that the tree cannot be pushed over by a big wind. Wind is also a wood

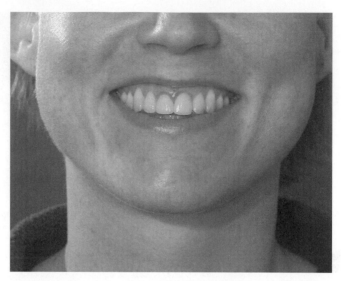

FIGURE 4-25.   The woman in this photo has a very strong jaw, which shows her determination, athleticism, and the desire to fight for what she believes in.

energy and means that other angry people cannot move you to change. Having shallow roots or a narrow jaw means the tree can be pushed over, uprooted, and moved. Individuals with a small jaw have trouble standing their ground. The jaw is measured best by the amount of bone below the ears. Jaws are certainly inherited but can also be grown. Although dentists hate me for saying this, grinding the teeth develops the jaw. Anger causes people to grind their teeth, but this anger is not necessarily expressed. Instead, it is directed at holding a position. Constantly grinding the teeth pulls the muscles over the jawbone, which irritates the bone and causes it to grow. The bigger the jaw, the more of a fighter a person is. This person has strong principles and ethics. People with strong jaws have determination and the ability to fight for what they believe in. These do not have to be correct beliefs, they are just strong beliefs, and they will hold them even if you try to convince them otherwise. You can count on people with big jaws to live by their principles and ethics and to keep their word.

An overdeveloped jaw indicates a tendency toward domination and dictatorship. Individuals with this type of jaw try to force others to believe as they do. They believe that their way is the right way; they often believe it is the only way. This is the jaw of a pugilist, someone who enjoys fighting, even for a living.

A narrow jaw (Figure 4-26) belongs to people who have situational ethics. They can be swayed by emotions because they are so pulled by the emotional content of the story. They can be influenced by persuasion. They prefer evaluating every situation based on the circumstances rather than from preconceived beliefs.

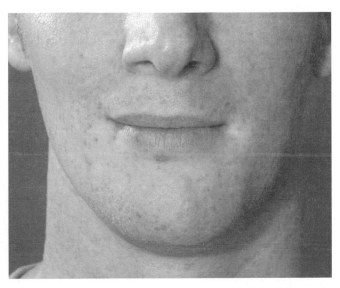

FIGURE 4-26.   The man in this photo has a narrow jaw, which means that he evaluates circumstances rather than holding preconceived ideas and beliefs.

Although they can change their minds based on new information, they are more likely to look at each situation separately. These people use more emotion in their decisions. That leads us to the fire element, the element that is most involved with feelings and the expression of emotion.

5 / *The Fire Features and Traits*

"Bright-flaming, heat-full fire, the source of motion."
Du Bartas, *Divine Weekes and Workes*

The strength of fire is shown in the eyes, the tips, and the corners of all the features and in every marking on the face. The fire element rules the heart. The heart is considered the emperor of the body. As the emperor, the heart rules the expression of all emotions. Even though every organ has its own emotions, the heart decides whether the emotion is to be expressed and how much it should be expressed. The fire element governs communications of all kinds, especially the use of words spoken verbally or in sign language with the hands. Because the heart controls expression, the wrinkles on the face show how much expression has been used over time.

The ancient Chinese had a fear of fire and were always recommending ways to contain it. Fire can be a dangerous element when overused because it dries up the *jing* and wears out the body. However, fire is also so necessary to the enjoyment of life that containing it too much may be even more harmful. There is a primal human need for expression and enjoyment.

The emotions that are particularly associated with the heart are joy and sadness. Practitioners of Chinese medicine today often talk of "excess joy" being dangerous. I believe that this is a mistranslation. What the ancients really meant was that excess excitement or mania, not joy, was considered harmful to the health. Also, sadness is often classified as one of the lung emotions. However, I believe that sadness is just the letdown from the high that fire lives on. It is the period between the time when the candle flame blows out and when it is relit. Because the heart and lungs are so connected, sadness can turn into sorrow, which is definitely a lung emotion. It then turns to grief, the primary lung emotion. People with lots of fire are fun, lively, charming, cute, and playful. They are expressive and changeable. The feature that is most closely associated with the fire element is the eyes because they are the best at showing emotion. Because of the complex network of muscles that surround the

113

eyes, they are the most expressive feature on the face and the most easily marked. We learn very early in life how to communicate with our eyes. They reveal our silent language. This is why eyes are so fascinating.

The fire element rules the firing of the brain's neurons, the synapses, and the receptor sites. One of the most important aspects of the fire element is the light of the eyes called the *shen*. By watching the *shen*, you can determine how quick someone's mind is by watching the alertness of the eyes. Babies with bright eyes are recognized as very intelligent. Fire minds can be so active that they never shut down, and this leads to some elaborate and active dreams. The *shen* shows the changes in emotion from moment to moment, and this light also shows how well the nervous system is functioning. The eyes tell everyone all about us.

EYE SIZE

Eyes tell our secrets. They are probably the most important feature on the face. The size of the eyes has always been correlated to the openness of the heart. Determining eye size is more of a subjective judgment than a measurement. Eyes are measured in terms of vertical height and must be viewed in proportion to the rest of the face. The genetic size of the eyes is not as important as how open people hold their eyes. People born with large eyes who deliberately narrow their eyes are suppressing their fire energy. When people have narrow or small eyes but hold their lids open, they are attempting to be more expressive and receptive. It is the amount of iris that shows that counts. You have the ability to determine the openness of your eyes within the boundaries of your genetic structure.

People with large eyes are emotional and have lots of fire energy. They have trouble controlling their emotions because they feel so much. They are reactive and expressive. They tend to feel before thinking and emote easily. Their emotions do not run as deeply because they let them out so easily. However, they are dramatic about their feelings and, while feeling them, believe that this is the way they will always feel. Their emotions change quickly, and they absorb other people's emotions. They tend to become infatuated quickly and are spontaneous and affectionate in public. They can be quite naïve and are easily disappointed.

Smaller-eyed people have a much better ability to control their emotions and, by doing so, push their fire energy into their brains. They have an active mental life and like to spend time calculating and planning. They think before they react, and they are much more logical and rational in their responses. They are often viewed as cold, but, in reality, they have deeper emotions that they have trouble letting out. They don't understand why other people don't realize how hard it is for them to express their feelings. Often when they think they have really let their emotions show, other people view their expression as tame. They are introspective and cautious. They tend to dislike public displays of emotion and are very private about their feelings. There is a natural tendency toward skepticism and distrust. They usually watch other people carefully. They do not fall in love easily, but when they do, they fall hard.

EYE SHAPE

Most people's eyes belong to one of five basic shapes, although each person's eyes will vary somewhat in terms of length and width. The most emotional and expressive kind of eye is called the *round eye*. These eyes are nearly as high as they are wide (Figure 5-1). People with these kinds of eyes have highly curved upper and lower lids, and nearly all of their irises show. These people are bold and gregarious and speak their minds easily. They are often childlike in their reaction to the world. They are constantly surprised and easily provoked emotionally. Round-eyed people are reactive and dramatic and tend to have intense mood swings. They have a tendency to go to extremes and possess a potential for recklessness. Usually short-tempered, they have an impudent charm that can soothe the ruffled feathers that they cause.

A variation of this eye type is simply called *large eye*. These eyes are still very big eyes and are rounded, but they are longer, and the lower lid is much straighter. Individuals with these eyes are expressive and artistic. They are usually very attractive to the opposite sex and are known to be romantics. They live by their emotions and tend to be impulsive. They are dramatic when angry and need to be creative to be happy. They dislike confinement and strict rules and live by their feelings. They have active imaginations and can enjoy their fantasy world more than real life when they have been hurt. They are very sociable and usually charming.

The opposite of this type of eye is called *little eyes*. Little eyes are much narrower and shorter but can be very cute (Figure 5-2). Individuals with these eyes are introverted and cautious. They hide their emotions from others and often from themselves. They have an extreme need for privacy in regard to their personal life and their feelings. They tend to scrutinize situations and other people, which encourages their suspicion of other people's motives. They are good with details and appreciate precision. They have a heightened sense of skepticism and do not trust easily.

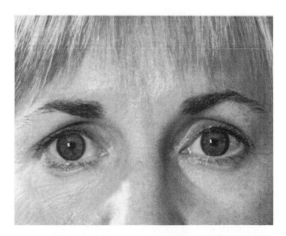

FIGURE 5-1.   The woman in this photo has round eyes, which is a sign of a bold and friendly personality. She most likely says what she thinks.

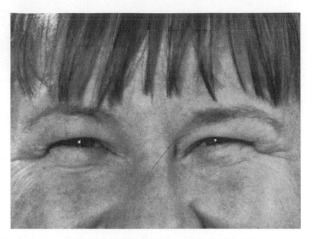

FIGURE 5-2.   The little eyes of this woman show that she hides her emotions inside. She most likely has a need for privacy and a feeling of trust in someone before she will reveal herself.

However, they are usually quite trustworthy and very good at keeping secrets. People with little eyes have a strong sense of reserve and are prone to a heightened sense of embarrassment when their feelings become known. They are much more comfortable in the thinking world than in the feeling one. And they think a lot.

The next eye type is called *almond eyes*. These eyelids curve slightly on the top and bottom. They still show most of their iris, but the height of the eye has been reduced. Almond eyes are longer than they are high (Figure 5-3). This is considered an exotic eye shape, primarily because it conveys a sense of mystery. A person with this type of eyes is very sensitive and warm but is not ruled by emotions. They exhibit caution about revealing deep feelings. They have more control of their

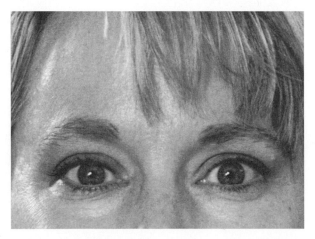

FIGURE 5-3.   The woman in this photo has almond eyes, which indicate strong emotions, but she has some reservations about expressing them.

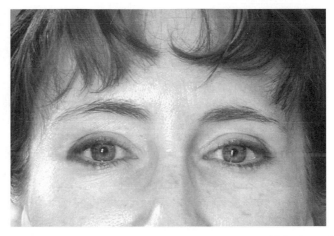

FIGURE 5-4. The woman in this photo has rectangular eyes, which show that she has an analytical mind. Although she has deep emotions, she is unlikely to express them easily, except for humor and anger.

emotions and can choose how best to express what they feel. They usually possess more common sense than people with larger eyes. They are viewed by most cultures as beautiful eyes and are also considered balanced. People with almond eyes are open enough to receive but cautious enough to analyze what they've gotten. They have strong emotions but evaluate when and how safe it is to express their emotions. They can vacillate between logic and feeling easily.

Rectangular eyes have eyelids that go primarily straight across the iris, and the eyes are long and narrow. This eye shape is much longer than it is high (Figure 5-4). This is also considered a balanced eye shape and is especially good for business. These eyes belong to thinkers. Their minds are more active than their emotions, and they are interested in using their logic rather than their feelings to deal with the world. They are not considered very emotional but, underneath the surface, can have deep passion. These people are difficult to get to know and to influence because they don't let much in. However, they are loyal to those they become close to and keep their friends for the long term. They are slow to make changes unless there is enough information to back up the decision. People with rectangular eyes are conscious of money and social status. They are often prone to envy. Emotions are usually held in, with the exception of anger, which is usually sharp and precise in its direction and target. These people can be perceptive about other people's motives.

EYE SET

The distance between the two eyes measures the set of the eyes. The average distance between the eyes is one eye length. If the eyes are spaced wider apart than that, you have a person with wide-set eyes. When the eyes are less than one eye length apart, you have close-set eyes.

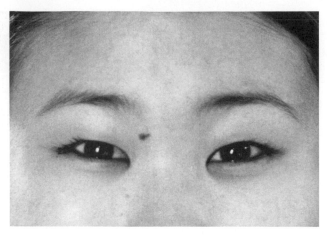

FIGURE 5-5.   The young woman in this photograph has what are often called *cat's eyes.* She is curious, clever, and changeable.

Wide-set eyes belong to people who are adaptable, flexible, and open-minded. They see life and knowledge with a broad perspective and usually dislike details. They can have trouble concentrating, but they tend to be innovative thinkers and tolerant of alternative views about life.

People with close-set eyes usually have keen powers of observation and are very analytical. They tend to focus on details and have less tolerance of views different from their own. Their perspective is sometimes narrow, but they have the ability to concentrate.

The slant of the eye is measured by determining whether one corner of the eye is higher than the other. If you were to draw a line from the inner corner of the eye straight across to the outer corner of the eye, the balanced eye would be level.

When the outer corner of the eye is higher than the inner corner, you have a person with an upturned eye (Figure 5-5). This type of eye belongs to curious and ambitious people. They are often referred to as *cat's eyes.* People with this trait can be opportunistic because they are quick to spot opportunities other people haven't seen yet. They also tend to be optimistic. They are entertaining, witty, and have clever minds.

A down-turned eye occurs when the outer corner of the eye is lower than the inner corner (Figure 5-6). These kinds of eyes are associated with sadness and soft-heartedness. These types of people are prone to pessimism and discouragement. They are often kind and compassionate but can be suckers for a sob story. They need to watch out for people who would take advantage of their softness.

EYE CORNERS

The inner corner of the eye is technically called the *inner canthus.* In face reading, it is an area that corresponds with the ability to use words, especially words used in

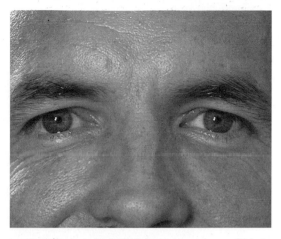

FIGURE 5-6.   The man in this photo has kind down-turned eyes. This is a sign of a soft heart and the ability to feel the sadness of others easily.

anger. The correlation is simple: the sharper the corner, the sharper the tongue. When the inner canthus is rounded (Figure 5-7), it signifies a person who is tactful and chooses words carefully. However, they can prevaricate and beat around the bush so much that their intent can be lost. When the inner canthus comes to a point (Figure 5-8), it indicates a person who uses words with great accuracy. Unfortunately, when people who have this trait get angry, the words can hurt. They are very carefully chosen and they are speaking truth—even if the truth is not very nice. When the corners point and curve downward (Figure 5-9), you have a person who uses words as a weapon. People who have this trait are very aware of it and usually try to do everything they can to resist using this trait. They know their sharp words can cause great emotional pain. Ironically, these people are usually very

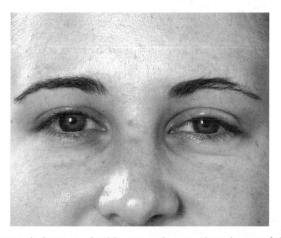

FIGURE 5-7.   The rounded corners in this woman's eyes show her tactfulness and care with words. She does not want to use words to hurt other people's feelings.

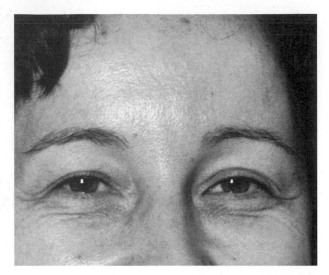

FIGURE 5-8.   The inner canthus of this woman's eyes comes to a sharp point, which indicates her ability to choose words very carefully but also tells of her sharp tongue when she gets angry.

sensitive and use this weapon only as a last resort. They pull out this trait when they feel they have no other choice because they are backed up against the wall. They go for the jugular and intend to inflict harm with their words. They are very focused in anger, perhaps more so than at any other time in their lives. Although they

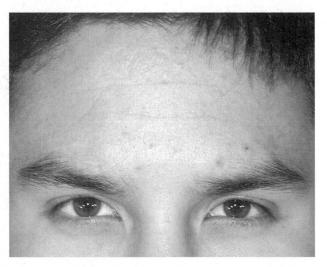

FIGURE 5-9.   The sharp and curved corners of this young man's eyes indicate the ability to use words as weapons. He chooses words precisely and for their emotional impact. This trait will rarely be seen by anyone except those closest to him, and only when they have caused him serious pain.

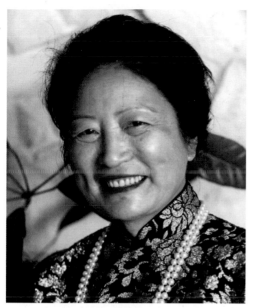

Color Plate 1: Mary C. Lowe. My grand-mother was a small, regal, and serene woman with a delightful giggle. Because of her wisdom, her beautiful face remained remarkably unlined despite the traumas in her life.

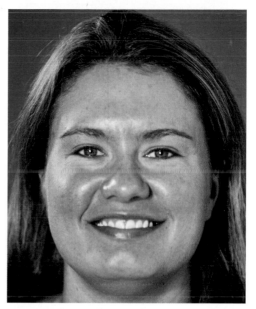

Color Plate 2: Square Face Shape. This is a woman with a lot of physical strength and stamina. Her squared jaw indicates leadership ability.

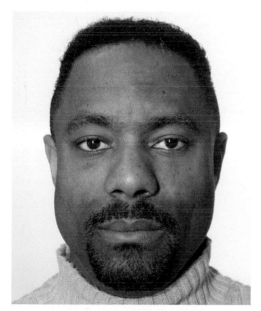

Color Plate 3: Rectangular Face Shape. This is a man with the subtle power that comes from a squared jaw in a longer face. He has manage-ment ability and the potential for promotion in business.

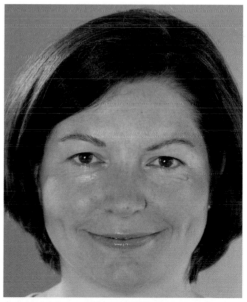

Color Plate 4: Round Face Shape. This is a woman with a friendly face, which is enhanced by her charming dimples. She is a natural sales-woman and deals well with people.

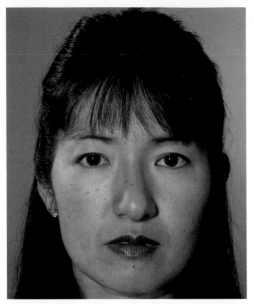

Color Plate 5: Oval Face Shape. This is a woman with an oval face, which indicates the graciousness of her hospitality. She is a peacemaker who wants everyone to get along and most likely has wonderful manners.

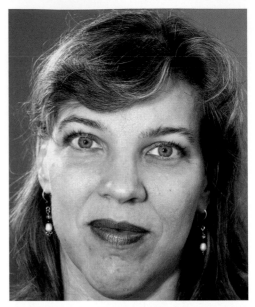

Color Plate 6: Triangular Face Shape. This is a woman with a creative mind with the focus that the triangular face shape embodies. The narrowness of her face also indicates her need to be alone.

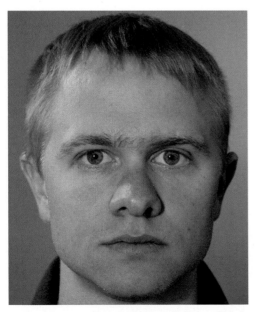

Color Plate 7: Trapezoid Face Shape. This is a man who has an inventive mind and an expressive personality. The breadth of his forehead indicates the expansiveness of his thinking, and the width of his face shows his desire to share what he comes up with.

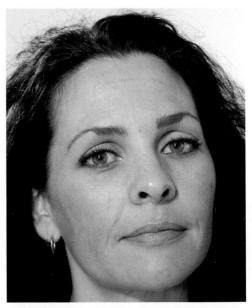

Color Plate 8: A Water Face. The deep and mysterious eyes are the strongest clue to the watery nature of this woman's personality. In addition, she has strength of bone structure, especially in her chin and upper forehead, which shows the dominance of her kidneys.

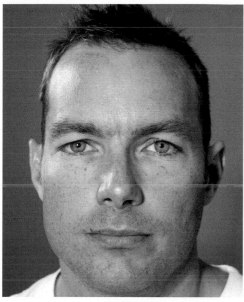

Color Plate 9: A Wood Face. This man's great eyebrows and very strong jaw are the clearest signs of a wood personality. The direct and focused gaze is another strong clue that shows his determination and athleticism.

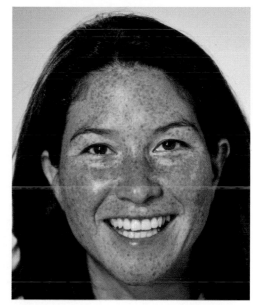

Color Plate 10: A Fire Face. This woman's charming freckles are the biggest giveaway to her fiery personality, but the sharp corners of her eyebrows, eyes, and mouth add fuel to the fire. Even more important is her big smile and the brightness of her eyes, which show she's a lot of fun!

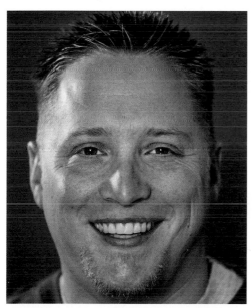

Color Plate 11: An Earth Face. This is a nice man with the generosity of earth as shown by his wide mouth and full lips. In addition, he has the beginnings of moneybags in his cheeks and a look of kindness in his eyes.

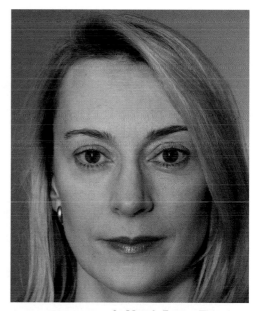

Color Plate 12: A Metal Face. This is a woman with all the signs of refinement evident on her face. She has an aquiline nose, delicate bone structure, high eyebrows, and a sculpted mouth. She looks expensive, as only metallic people can, and undoubtedly well worth it.

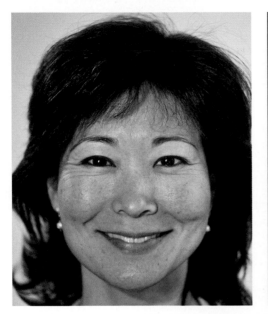
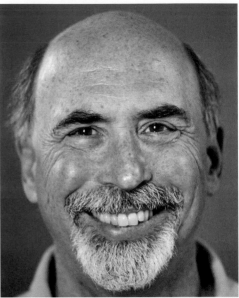
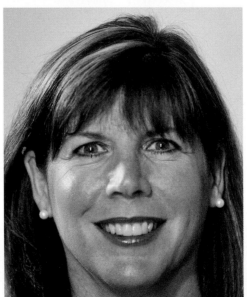

Color Plate 13: Significant *Shen*. These three people all have very bright *shen*. They are lit from within and have no problem expressing through their eyes.

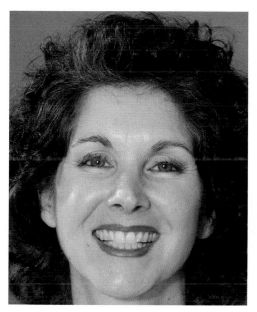 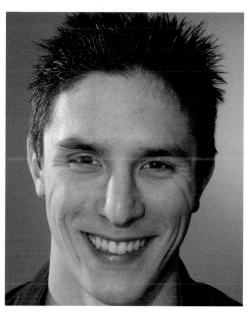

Color Plate 14: Sparkling Peach Luck. Electric smiles and sparkling eyes show just how contagious sparkling peach luck can be. This woman is excited about being alive and happy, and the high ears on this young man show a potential for fame, especially with this kind of peach luck so evident.

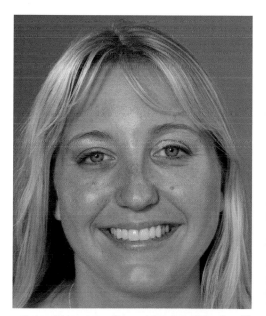 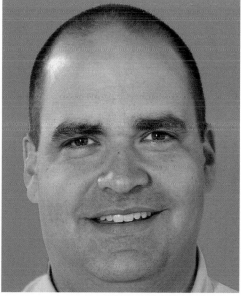

Color Plate 15: Supportive Peach Luck. The softness of these people's smiles and the warm glow in their eyes show how attractive supportive peach luck is. The woman is a romantic and loves to love and be loved, and the man is someone who has a good sense of humor combined with a good heart and generous spirit.

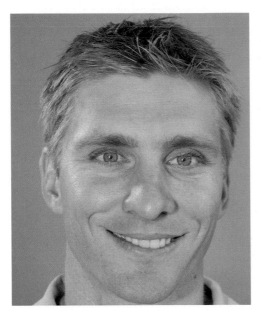
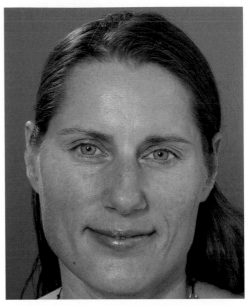

Color Plate 16: Dreamy Peach Luck. These two individuals are visionaries. All you have to do is look into the ethereal and translucent quality of their *shen* to be drawn into their dreamy peach luck. The man looks into the future and plans for a better world. The woman is an idealist and knows how it should be despite what she's seen.

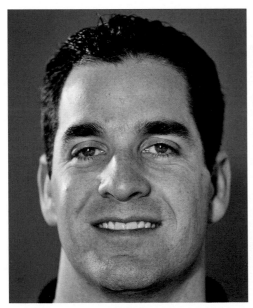
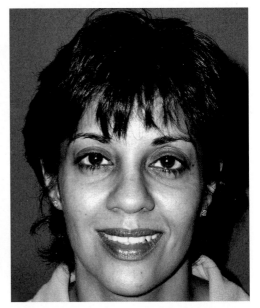

Color Plate 17: Seductive Peach Luck. Mysterious eyes and subtle smiles show the magnetism of seductive peach luck. This man is a little secretive but very deep and provocative. The woman shows wisdom in the depth of her eyes and the mole on her chin. Though hard to get to know, they already know about you.

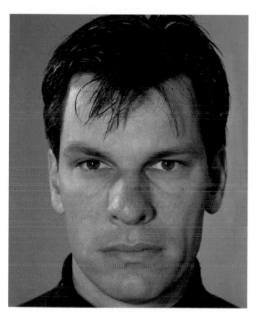 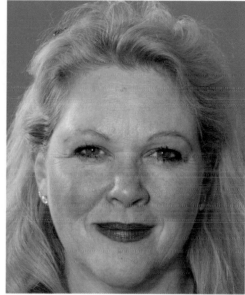

Color Plate 18: Direct Peach Luck. These two embody the mesmerizing qualities of direct peach luck in the fire and focus of their gazes. They don't even need to smile because they know what they want and how to get it. If you choose to go with them, it will be a very interesting journey. But you know who'll be in charge, don't you?

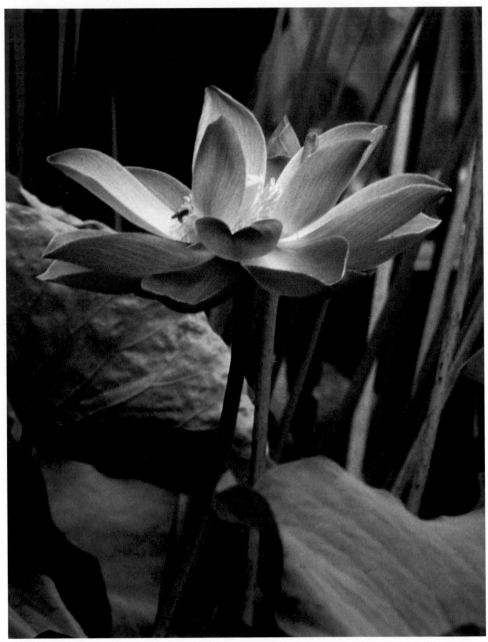

Color Plate 19: Lotus Flower. The lotus is an ancient symbol of purity, creativity, and beauty that rises upward, away from the attachments of the world, yet still a part of the world. Likewise, the lotus grows in the mud and water, and yet no mud or water can cling to the exquisite blossom. The lotus opens to bring beauty and light out of the darkness.

usually regret the pain they cause, the emotional wounds they inflict are usually not easily forgiven. This trait is most often used at the end of relationships.

IRIS

The iris is the colored portion of the eye that surrounds the pupil. The actual color of the iris is hereditary. The ancient Chinese were fascinated by variations in the color of the iris, primarily because most of their population had dark irises. They therefore looked at the richness of the color as well as the color of the light that comes off the iris, which is called the *shen* color. The Chinese believed that lighter-colored irises belonged to more mental people and that darker-colored irises indicated emotionality and passion. They believed that the color of the *shen* was the color of a person's spirit.

The best way to evaluate the color of the irises is to look at them in bright sunlight or with a strong flashlight. You are looking for the combination of colors that you see off the surface of the eye. For example, if someone has blue eyes with yellow flecks, it is very likely that the light coming off the eye is not blue. It may be aqua or some variation of green. Blue eyes are often seen as having gray *shen*, and brown eyes can have *shen* that varies from gold to orange. The *shen* color can be seen approximately ¼ inch off the eye.

Blue *shen* indicates a very mental person who can often be called *intellectual*. Aqua *shen* is correlated to idealists. Gray *shen* is tied to deep thinkers, whereas green *shen* is seen as mysterious with emotional depth. True brown *shen* belongs to friendly people. Gold *shen* indicates a mercurial temperament with enhanced magnetism. Any shade of red or orange in the *shen*, including rust and copper tones, belongs to people who are passionate and volatile.

WHITE-SIDED EYES

It is normal for the irises to be covered by a small portion of both the upper and lower eyelids. Eyes in which the whites show either below or above the iris are referred to as "three–white-sided eyes." This is an unusual manifestation of severely deficient fire energy. People who have three–white-sided eyes have an overactive nervous system and depleted adrenal glands. This overuse of fire energy creates nervous, hypersensitive, and edgy people. People with these kinds of eyes often complain of insomnia despite the fact that they are exhausted.

The most common form is three–white-sided eyes in which the white shows on the bottom, which the Japanese call *sanpaku*. In this case, the irises do not touch the bottom eyelid, and the whites of the eyes show beneath. Many ordinary people under severe stress or who are very sick have this trait. People with this trait can step on other people's toes because they are so reactive emotionally. They are temperamental, take offense easily, and are prone to making enemies. Three–white-sided eyes are not considered a dangerous trait when the average person manifests them. It can be a temporary condition caused by depression, illness, or exhaustion. It is a clear sign that the individual needs some serious rest and rejuvenation to calm down and reenergize. Such a person needs to learn to stop living on nervous energy.

Three–white-sided eyes in a famous person is considered a very dangerous trait that often leads to assassination (Figure 5-10). Famous public figures with this trait who were assassinated include Abraham Lincoln, Martin Luther King, Jr., John F. Kennedy, Yitzhak Rabin, and John Lennon. Even Princess Diana had this trait, and she was hunted by paparazzi, who were implicated in her accidental death. For years, I tried to determine why this trait was so dangerous in famous people.

In analyzing the assassinations, I realized that a person with severe psychosis or schizophrenia killed each of these famous people. Schizophrenia is correlated to

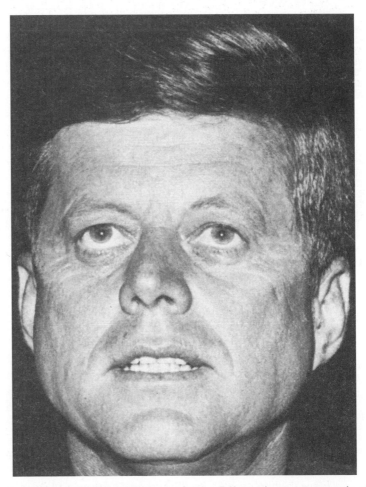

FIGURE 5-10. The three–white-sided eyes of John F. Kennedy are apparent in photographs of him even when he is younger. This trait was caused by his Addison's disease, or adrenal deficiency. However, it may also have contributed to his assassination.

misfiring in the brainstem, or the animal brain. This part of the brain is involved in instinct and impulse control. Three–white-sided eyes are a classic symptom of adrenal deficiency in all animals. In pack animals, a younger and healthier male will attack and kill a leader who shows signs of physical weakening. In misguided human beings, this same trait may be read and interpreted through their psychosis and paranoia. Unfortunately, the rigors of a famous life often lead to adrenal deficiency, giving many world leaders and celebrities three–white-sided eyes, which call out to the primal animal instincts of their would-be assassins. The assassins stalk and kill the leader or celebrity they obsess about in the delusional hope of gaining control and taking his or her place.

Three–white-sided eyes on the top is much less dangerous. It occurs when the upper eyelid does not touch the top of the iris. This gives someone the appearance of always being surprised or startled. In actuality, it is a sign of an overactive or even hyperactive nervous system that creates feelings of anxiety or panic. People with this trait are prone to hysteria because they are so tightly wound. It can also be a sign preceding violent behavior and will show just before the person snaps. People with upper three–white-sided eyes take everything personally and are hypersensitive to criticism or perceived attacks. If they do not have the energy to contain their fear, they can spin out of control.

The most severe form of white-sided eyes is four–white-sided eyes. This is a rare characteristic in which the iris is completely surrounded by sclera and both the lower and upper lids fail to meet the iris. People with this trait are unnaturally tense and prone to maladies of the nervous system. The ancient Chinese considered it a sign of a shortened life span because these people deplete their *jing* by living with so much fire. The blessing of this condition is that these people often have unusual minds, often bordering on genius. They have quick and sharp reactions. They are accident-prone and have overly active brains and excitable nervous systems. If their nervous energy is uncontrolled, it can lead to mental illness and manic behavior. Their eyes are opened so wide that they take in too many stimuli. They need to learn to shut out the world and live on a more balanced frequency.

TIPS AND CORNERS OF OTHER FEATURES

Fire marks every other feature on the face. Its flame touches and scorches the face, changing the landscape by the markings it leaves behind. Most of these markings are the lines caused by expression and past experience, but some markings occur when the fire element overacts on another element. Then the tips and corners of the features associated with other organs are kissed and singed by fire.

Ears that are pointed have been touched by fire. This is a sign of a person who has a tendency toward extreme emotions. The character Mr. Spock on the television show *Star Trek* had extreme examples of these kinds of ears. He was known for his lack of emotion, or what was eventually discovered to be his control over his emotions. After many years of *Star Trek,* there was finally an episode in which he lost control, finally revealing the true meaning of that trait.

Another fire marking of the ear has to do with the horizontal lines that cross the earlobe. In Western medicine, this trait has been tied to heart disease. However, in Chinese medicine, it is a sign of variable blood pressure, either too high, too low, or both. Blood pressure is certainly implicated in heart disease, but to the Chinese, this was by no means a direct marking for such problems.

When the fire element touches the eyebrows, it burns down the intensity of the wood element. Fire is shown in the tapering outside ends of the eyebrows. This is a sign of artistic ability and a strong sense of esthetics.

An unusual type of fiery eye is called the upside-down eye. This can be seen when you turn a photograph upside down and the eyes still look normal. It is a sign of a person who flips or makes 180-degree changes in opinions, ideas, or life-style choices. Individuals with this trait have a strong streak of unpredictability, as there is no way to know when they will make the switch.

Fire on the nose is shown on the tip. This area has one of the strongest correlations with the heart. One of the easiest things to see is a vertical line that bisects the nose between the nostrils. This is a sign of hereditary heart deficiency. Children with this trait are susceptible to heart murmurs. When the line cuts across the tip of the nose (Figure 5-11), this condition continues into adulthood and is correlated with mitral valve prolapse. Mitral valve prolapse has recently been determined to be a glitch in the nervous system, not a heart valve defect. Dr. Phillip Watkins, the director of the Mitral Valve Prolapse Center in Birmingham, Alabama, calls this syndrome *dysautonomia,* in which the glitch in the nervous system leads to low blood volume and the correlated feelings of dizziness, heartbeat irregularities, chest pain, panic attacks, and fatigue. According to Dr. Watkins, this disease affects up to 12% of the population, especially women.[1]

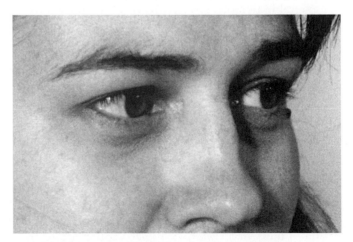

FIGURE 5-11.   The line that crosses through the tip of this woman's nose is indicative of fire deficiency or blood deficiency, which would cause fatigue and occasional hyperemotionalism.

[1]Roach M: A quick fix for fatigue, *Health* Oct, 1998.

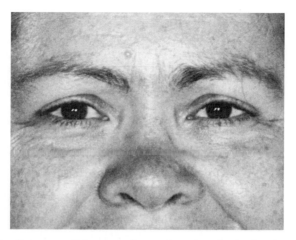

FIGURE 5-12.   The line across this woman's nose is a sign of a broken heart caused by some traumatic experience in the past. It has made her more cognizant of the bittersweet quality of life.

Another line cuts across right above the tip of the nose and is horizontal and signals an emotional fire deficiency (Figure 5-12). This is a sign of an emotionally broken heart in the past. A milder version of this is shown when the nose is upturned (Figure 5-13). This indicates a sentimental person. People with cute upturned noses are very sensitive and cry at sad movies, save souvenirs, and often make scrapbooks. They don't take any kindness for granted because they have been hurt in the past.

A turning down of the tip of the nose indicates a person who is not easily fooled by others. These types of people tend to be shrewd about others. Individuals in whom the nose tip covers part of the philtrum are also shrewd about finances.

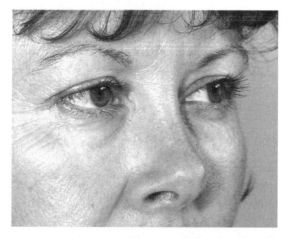

FIGURE 5-13.   The cute upturned nose on this woman's face is a sign of a sentimental person. She is probably very grateful for all kindness shown to her and cries at sad movies.

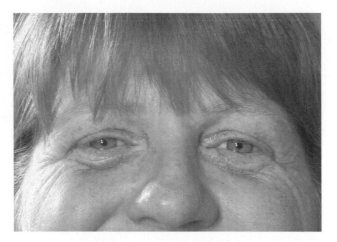

FIGURE 5-14. The rounded nose tip of this woman signals that she needs her creature comforts. She also loves being surrounded by beautiful things.

These people have hearts that are a little more closed down, and their minds are a lot more focused on business.

A rounded nose tip (Figure 5-14) belongs to a trusting person who needs creature comforts and pleasures. A squared nose tip (Figure 5-15) is indicative of a practical person. The nose tip is pointed in a person who has a "nose for news" (Figure 5-16). This person wants to find out why and get to the bottom of the mystery or solve the puzzle. They ask "why" a lot and collect information.

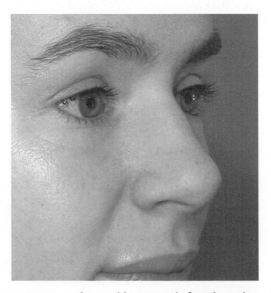

FIGURE 5-15. The square nose tip on this woman's face is a sign of a practical nature, especially when concerned with spending money. She wants nice things that have good value.

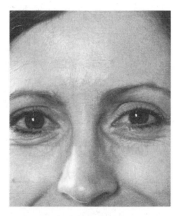

FIGURE 5-16. The tip of this woman's nose is pointed, which indicates her need to know why. She likes to get to the bottom of things and solve puzzles and mysteries.

The eyelashes are also a sign of fire energy. Thick, full, or long eyelashes belong to emotional and romantic people. Thin or straight eyelashes are found on a more pragmatic or realistic individual.

The corners of the mouth are directly tied to some important heart emotions. An upturned mouth (Figure 5-17) means a person is optimistic, cheerful, and positive, and this helps them attract attention. The down-turned mouth (Figure 5-18) indicates pessimism. People with this trait are prone to pessimism, often because of past disappointment.

The lip angles are also controlled by the fire element. People with lips that look as if they were etched and have sharp upper tips are very physically sensitive to stimulus. They dislike being tickled or treated roughly. They need gentleness because of their sensitivity. They hate being grabbed. Less defined lips belong to people who can take a rougher touch and enjoy a lot of tactile stimulation and even roughhousing.

When lines mark the middle of the lower lip, you have found a person who has a good sense of humor (Figure 5-19). These lines appear only if people laugh

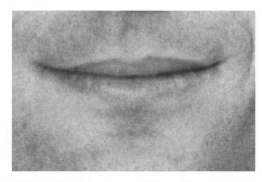

FIGURE 5-17. The lovely upturned corners on this man's mouth are a sign of his optimistic nature and his positive outlook on life.

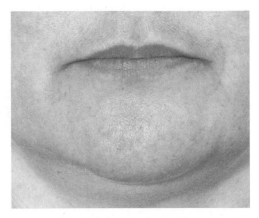

FIGURE 5-18.   The slightly down-turned corners on this woman's mouth indicate that she has been disappointed recently. This has made her view life with a little more pessimism.

or smile a lot, which causes their lips to stretch. The deeper the lines, the better the sense of humor. People with a few deep lines tend to appreciate slapstick humor or physical comedy. The lighter the lines, the more wit needs to be involved in the humor for the joke or story to be considered funny. This humor trait is emphasized by a dip in the lower lip. People with this indentation can find almost anything funny.

Dimples in the cheek (Figure 5-20) are one of the most attractive fire traits. They are a sign of extra magnetism and charm. Dimples allow people to get out of trouble easier because people who have them just look so cute! People with dimples

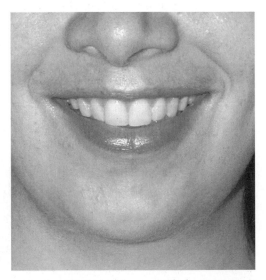

FIGURE 5-19.   The strong line through this woman's lower lip indicates her ability to be humorous as well as to enjoy humor from others. She laughs and smiles a lot.

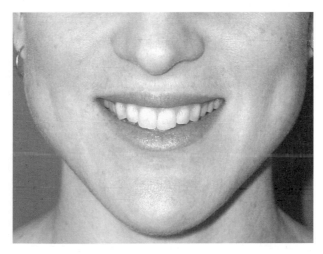

FIGURE 5-20.   The double dimples on this woman's cheeks give her lots of extra charm.

can get away with a lot and are forgiven easily. They are known to be glib and charming. However, the ancient Chinese cautioned that people with dimples could get away with using this trait only until they are in their midfifties. Then they have to do what they say and follow through.

A dimple in the chin (Figure 5-21) is a sign of a person who has a desire for attention, appreciation, and recognition. People with this trait need their thank-yous. They want you to pay attention to what they have done and to reward

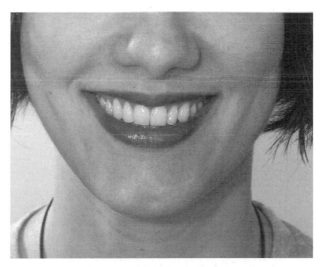

FIGURE 5-21.   This woman has a darling dimple on her chin and needs you to pay attention to her.

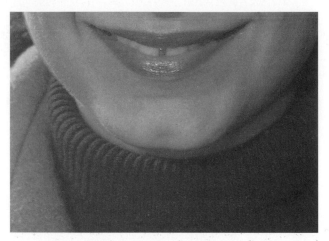

FIGURE 5-22.   This woman's cleft is a sign of the performer. She needs recognition and appreciation.

them accordingly. An individual with a cleft (Figure 5-22) is a natural performer. This was the child who always said, "Look at me!" As adults, they still crave the limelight. They want to be the center of attention and live for applause. Both the dimple and cleft belong to people who can end up being pleasers at their own expense. This is a classic case of fire (the dimple or cleft) overacting on water (the will). People with this trait would rather be liked than do what they are supposed to do. This trait is evident in the class clown. The attention becomes more important than the accomplishment. If you live or work with people who have this trait, be sure to tell them how wonderful they are all the time!

Fire energy is important because it makes life worth living. It's fun! People who have lots of fire energy can be charming and captivating or restless and annoying. Fire makes the mind more active and allows the emotions to be fully expressed. Without fire, life wouldn't be as vibrant or colorful. Like the flame, it appears in many forms. It flickers and roars, consumes and teases, entrances and changes. And, like the smoldering embers, it is always ready to be rekindled. The true meaning of fire is to experience all the variety that life has to offer. Fire is temporary and fleeting. To hold on to anything or stay connected, you have to go to the Earth element.

6 / The Earth Features and Traits

"How shall I celebrate the planet that, even now, carries me in its fruited womb?"
DIANE ACKERMAN, *THE PLANETS*

Earth is our home. We live on a planet of great abundance and amazing natural resources. Our earth nurtures us and provides all we need to survive and flourish. It is no wonder that tribal people around the world call our planet "The Great Mother." We are sheltered in her arms and fed by her bounty. Change is slow and constant on earth. Earth is our stability and the very foundation of our lives.

In Chinese medicine, earth energy is also the base element. It has to do with living in our bodies and feeling the pleasures of being human. Earth is concerned with feeding and nurturing the mind or body. Any problems of ingestion or digestion of either food or information is considered an earth condition. The earth element wants to take everything in, assimilate it, and make it part of the whole. It harmonizes discordant energies and is warm and embracing.

The earth element is most closely tied to the spleen and stomach. The stomach takes in a variety of foods, absorbs the nutrients, and transforms them into energy on which to live. The spleen breaks down old red blood cells in a different kind of digestion and helps fight infection. The earth element also corresponds to the pancreas and the ability to regulate blood sugar, the midback, the large muscles of the body, the lymphatic system, and the diaphragm. The earth element maintains the flesh of the body and is responsible for the amount of fat that is stored. The primary emotion of the earth element is worry, which leads to upset stomachs or confusion and a lack of clarity in thinking. Another major emotion of the earth element is sympathy. Earthy people feel great concern for those they love. They usually have a wide circle of friends and family members with whom they are involved. They enjoy being consolers and caretakers.

People with a large amount of earth energy have a soft plumpness to their bodies even when they are physically fit. This makes them cuddly! Because the earth element controls the large muscles of the body, when earth people are athletic, their bodies create very large, rounded muscles in the calves and biceps. Earth people tend to be slow moving, and they value consistency. They like to touch, such as in giving and receiving affection.

On the face, earth's strength is in the power of the features that correspond to the spleen and stomach. The mouth is considered the vital feature and shows the most information about the functioning of the entire digestive tract. Other features that correlate are the size and shape of the lips, the upper lip area, the bridge of the nose, the upper eyelid, and the lower cheeks. The earth element softens and rounds all the features of the face by putting an extra layer of fat around the bones. This creates cuteness and an ongoing resemblance to the faces of babies.

These earthy features show such traits as generosity, the desire for pleasure, the amount a person is able to give and receive, and the ability to accumulate. Earth people love their things and are great collectors. They are the gatherers and savers. The earth features are therefore considered the warehouses of the face.

THE MOUTH AND LIPS

The mouth is the place to take in nourishment and is also the most sensual part of the face. The size of the mouth shows the appetite. The bigger the mouth, the more a person wants. This relates not only to food but to affection and information as well. The mouth is a feature that expresses emotions easily, with a smile or a kiss. It is the second most changeable feature on the face, after the eyes. Most major expressions require movement of the mouth. The mobility of the muscles around the mouth allows people to change its shape and mark it. Unfortunately, most people press down on their lips and make them smaller.

The mouth shows generosity and the ability to give. Larger mouths (Figure 6-1) belong to people who have lots of earth energy. Mouth size is measured in relation to the nose. Create a triangle starting at the center point in the bridge of the nose and follow the sides of the nose down to the mouth area. The average mouth is the same length as the width at the base of this imaginary triangle. Any mouth that goes beyond this measurement is considered wide. A smaller mouth occurs when the corners of the mouth do not meet this distance.

To the ancient Chinese, a large mouth was considered a fortunate feature. Men with large mouths were supposedly more capable of getting a good wife. My great uncle spent a lot of time as a child trying to widen his mouth with his fist so that he would someday get a good wife. It worked. Perhaps because he was a generous man, he was able to bring out the best in his wife.

People with large mouths usually buy many presents for people they love as well as for business associates. They can be known to spontaneously give things even to strangers or new acquaintances. People with average-sized mouths still have generosity but are more particular about to whom and how much they give. People

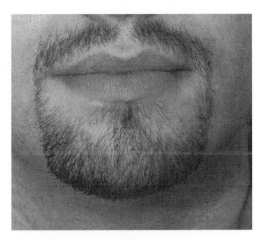

FIGURE 6-1.   This man has a large mouth that is indicative of a generous nature and strong earth energy. He gives easily and grandly.

with small mouths (Figure 6-2) find it difficult to give unless there is a good reason. They are more conditional about their giving. They give because someone deserves it or because they are supposed to give something and do so based on practicality more than emotion.

The size of the lips is also a factor. Fullness of the lips is evaluated based on the fleshiness of the rest of the face. Someone whose face is earthier, with plump cheeks and a puffy nose, will have bigger lips. Someone whose skin is taut with aquiline features will have thinner lips. Exceptions to this are *magnified traits*. In general, fuller lips belong to people who are more expressive emotionally. They are romantic and sensual. These lips indicate a desire for pleasure. People with thinner lips are more reserved emotionally, especially if they hold them compressed together

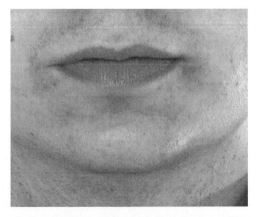

FIGURE 6-2.   This man has a smaller mouth, so he doesn't give quite as easily because he has less earth energy. The fullness of the lips, however, enhances his generosity.

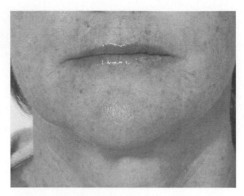

FIGURE 6-3.   The woman in this photo is holding her lips tightly together in a compressed way. This is a sign of suppressed emotions and a reserved person.

(Figure 6-3). This indicates a desire to hold their feelings in. They are proper and logical. They usually consider public expression of emotion to be unseemly. This does not mean that they are not romantic; they just save their emotional expression and romanticism for private occasions.

In the Western world, large lips are appreciated and valued on women. Because of this, many women spend lots of money buying lipstick to make their lips look bigger and lip gloss to make their lips look shiny and thus more prominent. Some get collagen and fat injections into their lips and even have GoreTex implanted. In men, however, thin lips are considered acceptable. Western men are expected to withhold expression of their emotions until it is appropriate. Thus men have learned to hold their lips tightly together. Many men have their lips compressed into a thin line. Westerners see this as a sign of a strong man who is in control of himself and his emotions. In actuality, it is a sign of repression and can lead to an inability to express. Men are expected to have a "stiff upper lip." This usually means that they don't have much of one at all!

People with wide mouths and full lips (Figure 6-4) express themselves easily in public and give easily to almost anyone, even people they barely know. They are

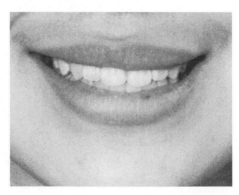

FIGURE 6-4.   This young woman has a generous mouth with full lips. These traits show maximum generosity and the ability to express emotions easily.

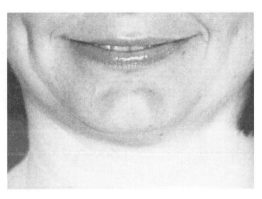

FIGURE 6-5. This woman with a wide mouth and thin lips doesn't express her emotions that easily but is generous, especially to those she loves. She is likely to give money or gift certificates.

spontaneous about giving and can be seen giving things away just because someone admired the objects. They get great pleasure from giving.

People with wide mouths and thin lips (Figure 6-5) are much more private about their feelings and don't express them easily. However, they do have an impulse for generosity and are most likely to give presents that are appropriate for the situation. They give to people deserving of a reward, or they give when it is the correct thing to do. They are the thoughtful business people who send out gifts to their customers at Christmastime and remember to send thank-you cards.

Small mouths with full lips (Figure 6-6) belong to people who express their emotions readily to those they trust and give generously to those they love. They reward loyalty and can use gifts to barter for favoritism. They are the people who look for exactly the right thing that their loved ones really want or need. This is often called the "Cupid's bow" mouth. They give for the pleasure of being loved and appreciated for their giving.

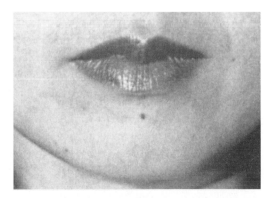

FIGURE 6-6. The small mouth with full lips on this woman indicate that she has strong emotions and the ability to express them to intimates. Her generosity is reserved for those who are close to her, and she is particular about what she gives.

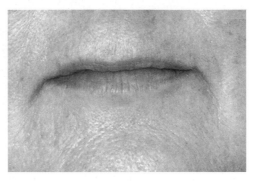

FIGURE 6-7. The small mouth with thin lips on this woman indicate that she gives most easily to those people whom she trusts completely. She has a harder time receiving than giving.

People who have small mouths with thin lips (Figure 6-7) have a little more trouble giving or expressing. They tend to be conditional about their gifts. People have to earn their gifts, or they give because they know that they have to. If the lips are held tight, it is a sign that these people have great self-control. They do not express easily or well and can appear to be lacking in warmth. Of course they do feel, but all feelings are kept hidden and out of view. They have great abilities to suppress emotions and hold onto money. If the lips are pinched, the bearer is a tightwad, both financially and emotionally.

When the lips are held tight in a pucker, you have found someone who is holding on to disapproval and resentment. You can bet that these people have followed the rules and done all the right things but somehow were not rewarded. Like a drawstring purse, they are capable of holding on to past hurts and resentment. Yet rather than being disillusioned by their lack of success, they usually believe that they were just unlucky. They can be judgmental because they still expect everyone else to follow the same rules even if those rules didn't work for them.

Sensuality and sexuality are also indicated by the size of the lips. Fuller, puffier lips belong to more sensual people. They enjoy experiencing life through their senses of touch, taste, and smell. They luxuriate in the pleasures of life and need to experience life this way. Although sensuality is often associated with sex, it does not have to be. People with full lips do not have a stronger sex drive. Their need for sensuality can be met in many ways. They love the feel of a creamy pudding or the softness of silk against their skin. They can usually find many ways to experience their sensuality, of which sex is only one aspect.

In contrast, people with thin lips usually have a stronger need for sexuality. They do not allow themselves much self-expression. They still have sensual needs and during sex is one of the few times they allow themselves to feel and express their sensuality. These kinds of people can be sensual lovers but don't touch much unless they are making love. They limit their intake of pleasure and put brakes on their expression. If the lips are held very tight, these people may have repressed their ability to be sensual at all.

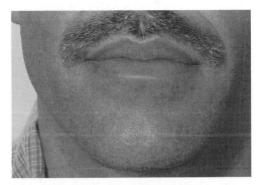

FIGURE 6-8. The man in this photo has an upper lip only slightly bigger than the lower. He is still dramatic about his feelings, however, and most likely is cranky as an invalid.

When the upper lip is larger than the lower lip (Figure 6-8), you have found a person who desires intense emotional experiences. Otherwise known as a "drama seeker," this kind of person takes all emotions to extremes. This is often seen when the upper lip has a little extra flesh in the middle that comes down over the lower lip. This kind of lip can also be found on men, and such men make the worst patients when they are sick or injured. They are sure they need stitches when they are cut, are convinced they are dying until they are diagnosed with the flu, and are positive they have broken something when it is just a sprain. They live life as though they were in an Italian opera and are prone to exaggeration and emotional flourishes. When down, they believe that life will always be this way and never get better. They can be very entertaining or very exhausting. The saying in Chinese is that these people would rather fight than be bored. This trait is exaggerated when the lip is very puffy.

If the upper lip is flaccid and remains open when the mouth should be closed, the bearer has poor boundaries. One of the corollary signs is gums that show easily. This is a trait more often associated with women who have weak morals and are easy prey both emotionally and sexually. Often a sign of previous sexual abuse, a woman with this trait is vulnerable to predatory people and lacks distinction between herself and others. Interestingly, many actresses and models try to emulate this look in photographs, thinking that it makes them look sexy. In reality, it makes them look needy and vulnerable to mistreatment. It is a sign of sexual or physical openness.

Some people have very big teeth that keep their lips from closing completely. Their lips are not large enough to close over the teeth, and they are usually very self-conscious about it. These are talkative people who make their lips thinner by trying too hard to hold their mouths shut. They need to relax and just be their outgoing selves. They are trying too hard to control their natural impulses to communicate. This kind of mouth belongs to people who are open emotionally and are likely to talk to strangers about personal things and feelings.

If the lower lip is fuller than the upper lip (Figure 6-9), the bearer desires physical pleasure. These people need to eat good food, drink fine wine, and sleep

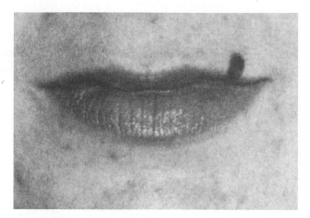

FIGURE 6-9.   The woman in this photo has a bigger lower lip, which indicates her desire for physical pleasure and comfort. The refinement of her mouth also shows that she has very good taste.

in comfortable beds. They do not tolerate discomfort and demand the best they can get. The fuller the lower lip, the more comfort and luxury this person needs (Figure 6-10). If the lip is also puffy, it is a sign of hedonism. People who have a protruding lower lip pout well when they don't get their way. This is a sign of self-indulgence. If the lower lip is considered lax and lacks tightness in muscle tone, you have found a person who has poor self-control and is prone to lasciviousness. These individuals have an inability to curtail the hedonistic impulses, which can get them into trouble in many ways. Problems with overindulging in both food and sex are correlated. This trait is more often found in men than in women.

In the ancient texts, men with this kind of lower lip were admonished to be careful not to have too many mistresses or they would die in financial ruin.

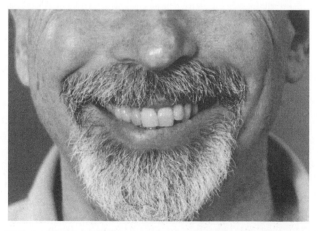

FIGURE 6-10.   This man's very full lower lip indicates that he is a gourmand. He loves good food, good wine, good company, and luxurious surroundings.

The ancients believed that a man with this trait would not be able to control his sexual desires. Therefore one woman, especially if she was his wife, was obviously not going to be enough. Considering how expensive mistresses were financially and energetically, these men were obviously doomed. Of course there are other traits that may curb these desires, but this trait is still considered a sign of poor impulse control and possible gluttony or addictive tendencies.

Individuals with lips that show firmness and strong muscle tone not only have good muscle tone in the digestive organs, especially the diaphragm and intestines but also have great discipline. Of course, they could also be called anal-retentive. When the lips are flaccid and loose, the digestive tract is also likely to have poor muscle tone, and the person has difficulty with retention. When the lips are puffy and dark, you have signs of digestive stagnation.

The area above the upper lip is one of the best areas for determining the functioning of the stomach, which is discussed later in terms of coloring. It is also the place to look for issues about nurturing. Because the earth element is so involved with the ability to give and receive, the upper lip area shows how well someone manages these desires. People with a strong earth element have a lot of extra nurturing to give, and this area is full. If the earth element is deficient or if someone gives away too much nurturing, the upper lip area is sunken and marked (Figure 6-11). Vertical lines in this area indicate overnurturing of others at the expense of oneself. Deep or numerous lines are a sign of other-directedness. These traits show overuse and a deficiency of the earth energy. People with these lines have worried too much about others and given too much of themselves away. Although these lines are associated with smoking, there is still an underlying need for self-nurturing that smoking seems to fulfill. These individuals smoke to help clear the mind of worry and therefore have the illusion of being nurturing to themselves. In reality, because smoking is fiery, it is sends smokers backward on the five-element cycle and is therefore destructive. The prescription for these lines is true self-nurturing, specifically luxury and pampering. This gets people going in

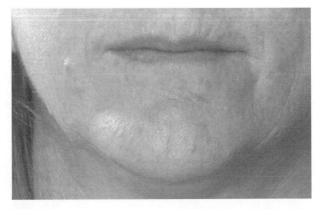

FIGURE 6-11.   The woman in this photo has multiple small lines in her upper lip, which means that she has overnurtured other people and undernurtured herself. She needs some pampering.

the right direction on the five-element cycle, from earth to metal. These kinds of behaviors increase self-esteem and self-worth.

BRIDGE OF THE NOSE

The area on the nose directly between the two eyes is a minor earth area. It is an area that correlates with the pancreas and shows blood sugar problems. Small lines here accompanied by a light or white color indicate low blood sugar or hypoglycemia (Figure 6-12). Strong lines or darkness in the area is a sign of excess blood sugar or the tendency toward diabetes. In babies, this area is often blue. This is a sign of blood sugar irregularities in the baby. It is usually a direct reaction to the mother's diet or a reaction to formula. Babies with this marking often have food intolerances and allergies and are prone to colic.

UPPER EYELIDS

In Chinese medicine, puffy upper eyelids are a sign of earth excess. This trait is also associated with spleen dampness, where the dam of earth keeps the water contained and stagnant. This contributes to weight gain and obesity. The emotional correlate is that these kinds of people do not suffer for love and never lose their appetite. People with puffy upper eyelids (Figure 6-13) are also supposed to be very good at saving money and investing it, especially in real estate. When the upper eyelid is sunken, hollow, or deeply lidded (Figure 6-14), the bearer suffers easily and often. When they are upset, they do not eat or sleep and lose weight and money easily. This is a sign of earth deficiency because they have trouble holding onto things, including their energy, when they are suffering.

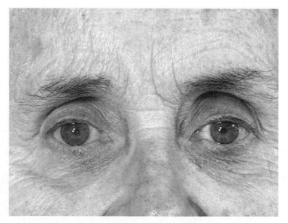

FIGURE 6-12.   The woman in this photo has lines in the bridge of her nose, and the area is lighter than other parts of her face. This shows a tendency to be hypoglycemic and also the need to nurture herself through her diet.

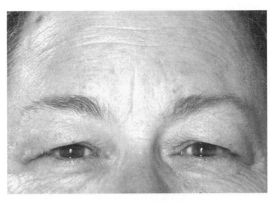

FIGURE 6-13. The woman in this photo has puffy upper eyelids, indicating that she has slight spleen dampness but also has the ability to save money and invest in real estate.

LOWER CHEEKS

The last area of earth energy on the face is the area of the lower cheeks, also known as "moneybags" (Figure 6-15). This area is the fleshy part of the face above the jaws, often called *jowls*. To the ancient Chinese, this was one of the most important areas of the face. It was considered the primary warehouse of the face and showed whether someone could accumulate reserves of energy or money. It was important to have moneybags before you even got the money. And if you got rich or had extra energy, the moneybags were sure to show up. It was also cautioned that this area should not look "like mutton fat jade," which meant cold, hard, and white. That was a sign of grasping materialism and would lead to severe health problems caused by excess earth. Instead, this area should look like the skin of a white peach, with a pale rosy blush, firm but soft and full. If the skin sags here, it is a sign of depleted earth energy.

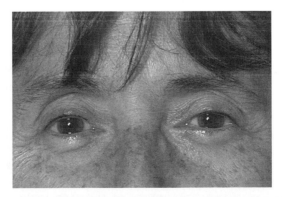

FIGURE 6-14. The woman in this photo has suffered in the past, probably because of a lost love, as seen from the strong lines under her eyes. She undoubtedly takes on the suffering of others as well.

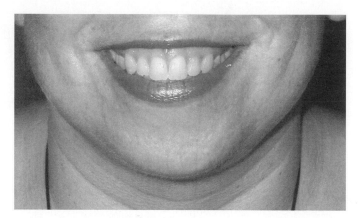

FIGURE 6-15. The lovely moneybags on this woman's face are a sign of extra earth energy and show her ability to save money and energy. This is the most important warehouse on the face.

Moneybags were a signal that a person could withstand a famine because they had just enough extra weight to live off of for a while with enough extra energy to find more food. Too much extra weight meant that someone was too sedentary and would be unable to mobilize to find food and would be too slow to seize future opportunities. Too little weight on the body would mean that a person could starve to death too easily and had nothing left in reserve for recovery.

The ancient Chinese also considered any long-term disease that caused great pain or illnesses, like influenza, a famine condition. When people have a disease that causes wasting or chronic pain, they lose energy and strength to fight for their survival. They are also incapable of keeping on weight that buffers them from pain. Illnesses such as the flu with a high fever eliminate the desire to eat and keep the body from recovering as quickly. Food was and is one of the best sources of energy replenishment. The ancient Chinese believed that people with moneybags would be able to survive the critical first days or weeks of a famine and then still have enough energy left to regroup and recover. They recommended that healthy people keep an additional 10 pounds of surplus fat on their bodies.

Moneybags and the extra 5 to 10 pounds they imply are no longer considered as attractive, because we value a thin vision of beauty over optimal health. However, moneybags are also a sign of people who are living life slowly enough to feel, enjoy, and relate to others. These are people who know what gives them pleasure, and they also know how to receive it. They have the ability to accumulate enough things or money or friends to feel rich. As in the old saying, "It takes money to make money," people with moneybags attract more because they have something extra already.

The minor warehouses of the face include plump earlobes (Figure 6-16), which belong to the water element, but the earth element adds the ability to hold onto investments that ensure financial security in old age and luck in

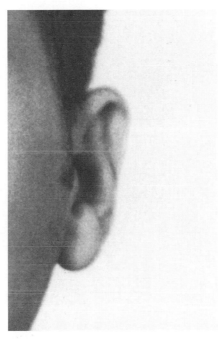

FIGURE 6-16.   This man's earlobes may be small, but they are plump. This is a sign of the ability to invest for the long term, with eventual reward in old age.

acquiring and keeping real estate. This is like an earthen dam that helps hold the water energy in and encourages accumulation. A plump chin (Figure 6-17) is a sign of stubbornness. This is the equivalent of digging one's feet into the ground. Although the chin is part of the water element, the extra earth here blocks "going with the flow." A plump chin is also a sign of possible future weight gain, otherwise known as "spleen dampness." The earth element also adds plumpness to big cheekbones (Figure 6-18), which makes authoritative people

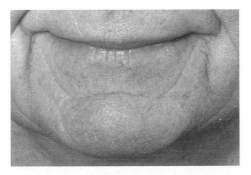

FIGURE 6-17.   The man in this photo has a plump chin that is also turned up. The plumpness and the turned-up quality double his trait of stubbornness. You can be sure he digs his heels in well and often.

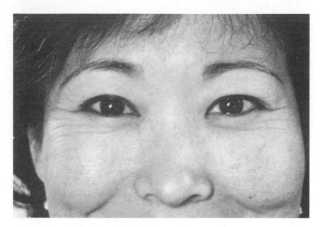

FIGURE 6-18. The woman in this photo has plumpness covering up strong cheekbones. She can be bossy in such a nice way that people may not even realize that they are being bossed around.

friendlier, because earth is much warmer and more people oriented than the metal element that controls the cheekbones. Earth energy helps round the nose tip, which shows an increased desire for material things and the ability to get them. This is another metal feature that gets softened by the earth element and helps people experience pleasure and comfort.

The original meaning of wealth was food, having enough grain (rice, wheat, barley, or millet) for your own family and enough left over so you could trade it for other food or things that made life more pleasurable and comfortable. This was a good, earthy life. Eventually, as societies became bigger and more complicated, barter was taken over by the use of money, created in the original form of metal coins. The metal element takes raw materials from the earth to create things of even more value, such as coins, jewelry, cutlery, and machinery. It creates treasures from the primitive and unformed. The metal element also creates the refined, aquiline features of the face.

7 / The Metal Features and Traits

"Metal is a refined extract of Earth forged by Fire"
DANIEL REID, *THE COMPLETE BOOK OF CHINESE HEALTH AND HEALING*[1]

The metal element is a challenge to understand. Although it is best symbolized by the Chinese coin, it also corresponds to the Western element of air. The correlation makes sense, because the ancient coin was solid but had a hole (or air) in the middle. The metal element is a dichotomy; it is the circle with the square within. It is composed of two colors of metal, warm gold and cool silver. It is substantial and yet ethereal. These seemingly contradictory aspects do not need to be blended. In fact, balancing the metal element involves being both things at the same time. It corresponds with breathing in and out. In Chinese medicine, the primary organ of the metal element is the lungs, which are the highest vital organ in the body except for the brain. The lungs are the organs most easily affected by external influences such as cold, heat, wind, bacteria, or viruses. The corollary parts of the body include the shoulders and the upper back, the colon, the bronchi, the mucous membranes, and body hair.

The vital feature of the metal element is the nose. The bigger, stronger, or more beautiful the nose is, the stronger the metal element is. The secondary metal features are the cheekbones, the upper cheeks, and the skin. The metal element is also responsible for the distance and space between the features. The emotions involved with this element are sorrow and grief. The issues are about the ego, boundaries, and the feeling of lack or plenty.

Any refinement of the features or bone structure indicates the influence of the metal element. Metal is the civilizing influence of the elements. It polishes rough edges, cuts away the unnecessary and irrelevant, and creates a buffer to protect from the harshness of the outside world. People with a lot of metal energy appear

---

[1]Reid D: *The Complete Book of Chinese Health and Healing*, Boston, Shambhala, 1995.

145

serene and calm. Their features often appear chiseled and precise. Very symmetrical or aquiline features indicate emotional strength of the metal element.

NOSES

The ancient Chinese correlated large noses with nomadic ancestors who came from very cold climates. Because the air was so cold there, people developed longer and larger noses to warm the air before it entered the lungs; otherwise the lungs would be damaged. Living in such hostile environments required having an ego that was strong enough to believe that you were supposed to survive under such conditions and gave these individuals the ambition to work hard to make life better. Therefore large noses (Figure 7-1) correspond to a healthy ego, and long noses to ambition. However, the effects of the climate could isolate people, so there is an implication of a large nose also implying the loner mentality and an independent spirit. A long nose was correlated to ambition and a drive to succeed despite obstacles.

As in all measurements on the face, the size of the nose needs to be correlated in relation to the size of other features and the size of the whole face. The fleshiness of the rest of the face and how it corresponds with the nose must also be evaluated. It is uncommon for someone with a narrow face and very narrow features to have a big, fleshy nose. However, it is possible and means even more because it is so unusual. Likewise, people with very wide faces and fleshy features are unlikely to have small or very narrow noses. If they do, they are breaking out of a pattern, and this is very important information about their personality and health.

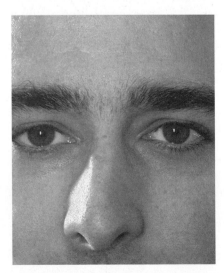

FIGURE 7-1. The man in this photo has a large nose, which indicates his ambition and his willingness to work hard to achieve his goals. He does have ego needs that can be filled only by a sense of accomplishment.

A large nose shows the potential for a large ego because it is symbolic of large lungs. The lungs are like a balloon: The more air you put into the balloon, the bigger the balloon gets. When people have puffed-up chests, it is said that they are "full of themselves" or that they are "full of hot air." In either case, it shows that people who feel good about themselves breathe in deeply and stand up straight, showing off their confidence. Likewise, when people have very little confidence, they hunch their shoulders, and their chest becomes concave. Chances are they also have a smaller nose. A large nose can also be a sign of power. Luckily, because the metal element is about ideals, the power is usually used for making the world a better place. This is also a sign of great individuality.

When someone has a small nose (Figure 7-2), it means that the person's ancestors came from a warm or tropical climate, where the air was very easy to breathe because it was warm and humid and food was plentiful. People living there didn't have to fight the elements to survive. People from these places were therefore believed to be more passive and group-oriented. They lived cooperatively and socially. It was deduced that play was very important for people with small noses.

People with little noses want to blend in, not stick out in a crowd. They need to spend a lot of time feeling as if they are playing; this is especially important in work. They prefer an easier life and a relaxed work atmosphere if they have to work. They often long for the good old days when life was less rushed and people were friendlier. They enjoy group activities and prefer being part of the crowd. They are not as personally ambitious.

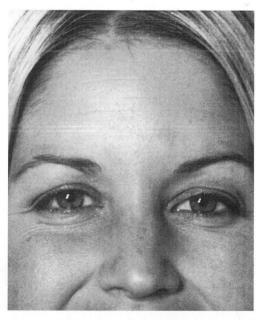

FIGURE 7-2.   The woman in this photo has a small nose, which shows her desire to have fun. Life will be most enjoyable for her when she feels as if she is playing or taking it easy.

When the nose comes off the face by over an inch (Figure 7-3), you have found a person who is a trailblazer. People with noses that protrude a great deal when in profile like to do things in a new and different way. They dislike routine and following the herd. They are pioneers and adventurers. When Western sailors first reached the shores of China, the Chinese were amazed at how large their noses were. In fact, their nickname for them was the "Big Noses." They were from northern European countries, and the Chinese were particularly impressed with how far off the face the noses protruded. This was a trait that was very rare in China and of course explained to them why the travelers would want to leave the safety of their homeland to come to a foreign place—it was all because of their noses!

Noses that are flatter belong to people who are content to live life as it has always been lived. They are slower to grasp innovation and change and prefer the old-fashioned to the newfangled. People with flatter noses are more conforming and much less adventurous. They are more likely to travel with someone else or in tours. They don't understand the draw of dangerous expeditions except to experience them vicariously. Someone else's adventure is close enough. They often have security issues and prefer the anonymity of groups. People with small noses are cooperative and work wonderfully with other people and within the family (Figure 7-4).

The nose has also been called the "moneybox of the face." The bridge of the nose shows how much money can come in or how much energy the bearer has to use. The base of the nose, including the nostrils, shows how much money or energy can be saved. A fleshy nose (Figure 7-5) is considered a sign of materialism. The earth element has added emphasis here and contributes the ability to appreciate and accumulate things. Individuals with this type of nose value having

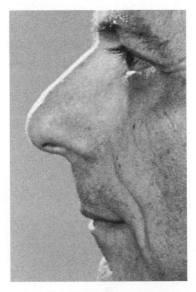

FIGURE 7-3.   The man in this photo is a trailblazer, as can be seen from his nose, which comes off his face. He likes to do things in a new and different way and sees himself as progressive.

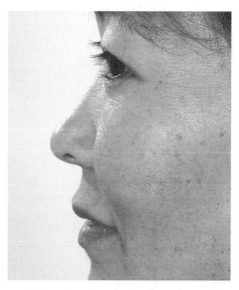

FIGURE 7-4. The woman in this photo is a cooperative, group-oriented individual. She does not need to stand out in a crowd. She prefers the achievement that comes from a group effort.

a lot of things. If the nose is bulbous, the bearer overindulges in the physical world and its pleasures. This kind of person accumulates simply for the joy of having large quantities of things.

Thin or narrow (often called *aquiline*) noses belong to people who value ideals over money (Figure 7-6). They care more about quality than quantity. They would rather have exactly what they want than manage with something temporary, so they will live without. A bony nose indicates a person who eschews material things and would rather live simply and like an ascetic. People like this often value a monastic-type existence and prefer hardship to pleasure.

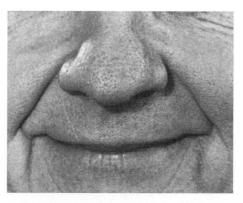

FIGURE 7-5. The man in this photo has a fleshy nose, which indicates the need for material pleasure. He enjoys accumulating and collecting.

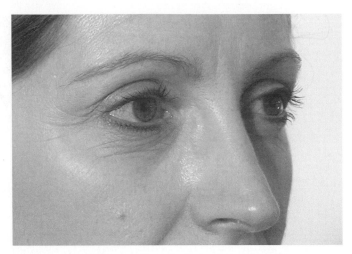

FIGURE 7-6.   The woman in this photo has a long, delicate nose that is often called *aquiline*. This means that she values ideals over things. She cares more about the quality or beauty of the things she has, rather than how much she has.

When the bridge of the nose is wide (Figure 7-7), it is a sign of extra energy for making money. Money comes in more easily and in larger quantities. When the bridge is narrow (Figure 7-8), there is less energy for working, and physical labor is out of the question. It is also hard for people with this type of nose to bring in large amounts of money at a time. Instead, money comes in small increments.

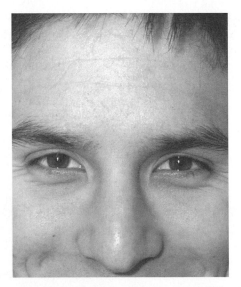

FIGURE 7-7.   The young man in this photo has a nose with a wide bridge. This indicates physical strength and stamina and the ability to make money in large amounts. In addition, it is a sign of a very strong spine.

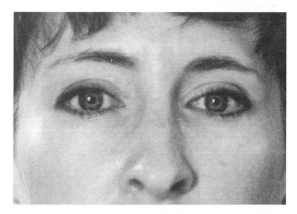

FIGURE 7-8. The woman in this photo has a nose with a narrow bridge. This is a sign of less physical energy, and money will be earned in smaller amounts. It also signifies a more delicate spinal structure.

A bump on the bridge of the nose (Figure 7-9) is a sign of someone who wants to be in charge. This is one of the signs of pride. This kind of person is not a good follower but makes a good leader. If the nose slopes and turns upward (Figure 7-10), the bearer is more of a follower. The work of this individual eventually pays off because the energy down the nose is said to come back to the person later in life.

Nostrils are the second part of the moneybox. They are like the hole in the piggybank that lets the money or energy out. Nostrils that are very wide indicate

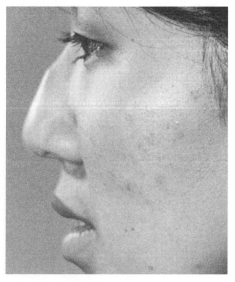

FIGURE 7-9. The woman in this photo has a nose with a bump on the bridge. The Chinese consider this protrusion a sign of a person who needs to be in charge. She is a leader, not a follower.

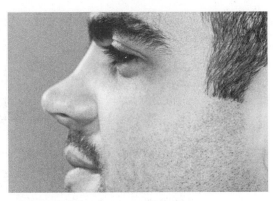

FIGURE 7-10.   The man in this photo has a nose that slopes downward and then tips back upward. This person follows direction well, and if he bides his time, he will attain success later in life, as money is supposed to come back to him in the end.

a person who spends energy and money easily. For these types of people, it's "easy come, easy go." Narrowed nostrils (Figure 7-11) are a sign of individuals who want value for their money. They still spend, but they are trying to save at the same time. Lots of people like this can be seen at warehouse super-stores buying large quantities of things because they are sold at a discounted price. These people also buy things on sale. In terms of energy, they look at different circumstances and determine the energy expenditure required. If spending their

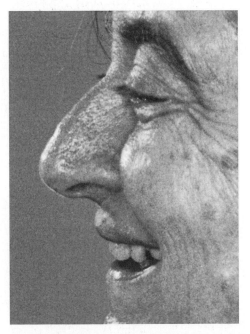

FIGURE 7-11.   The woman in this photo has long and narrow nostrils. Although she may enjoy spending, she wants value for her money and time.

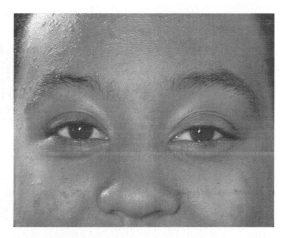

FIGURE 7-12.   The young woman in this photo has small nostrils, which means that she will evaluate how much things cost before she spends. She doesn't let go of money easily, and she has the ability to hold onto it well.

energy pays off later, they will use their energy. Small nostrils (Figure 7-12) indicate a person who holds onto money and energy. These people don't like to spend; however, this does not mean that they are cheap. They are just very aware of how much things cost. For example, if they have to go to a business party, they determine how long they will stay based on how tired they are going to be from having to make small talk. They are also very aware of how much energy it took for them to make the money that they are about to spend. Nostrils that are flared (Figure 7-13) are a sign of enhanced ability to smell as well as an increased need for buying things of esthetic value.

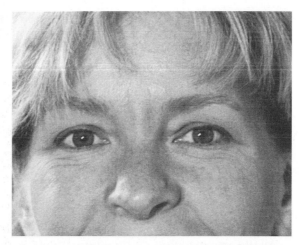

FIGURE 7-13.   The woman in this photo has nostrils that flare. This is a sign of a heightened sense of smell and enhanced esthetics. She has very good taste and won't spend her money on anything that isn't beautiful.

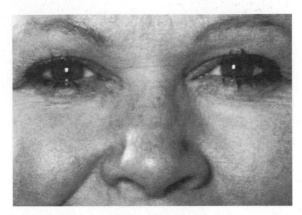

FIGURE 7-14.   The woman in this photo has very defined alae, or the flesh that surrounds her nostrils. This shows that she can be very disciplined about money and very good at saving it.

The alae, or sides of the nose that contain the nostrils, also add some emphasis to these traits. If the alae are very firm and well defined (Figure 7-14), the bearer is disciplined about money and can hold onto it. If the alae are looser and less defined, the bearer is more lackadaisical about personal routines and finances. If the alae are flat, there is a lack of discipline both personally and financially.

One of the more fascinating things about the nose is that it is a hologram of the spine. When someone has an injury to the spine, even a pulled muscle, you are able to see it on the nose. I have had students with scoliosis whose noses curved the same way as their back. A straight bridge of the nose shows proper alignment of the spine. The very top part of the nose between the eyes corresponds to the neck area. If this area is narrow, the structure of the neck is considered fragile. People with narrow bridges are prone to whiplash and can damage their necks easily in accidents. When the bridge is wide, the structure of the neck is solid and strong. The shoulders and upper back are represented at the end of the bone in the nose about one fourth of the way down from the bridge. If this area is broad, the person likely has broad shoulders. Narrowness here indicates narrow shoulders. If the skin is pulled in any way so that striations appear, you are looking at muscle problems in the upper back. The midback is represented halfway down the nose, where the underlying structure is cartilage. This area is right above the top of the alae. This is a very common place for the skin to be pulled, showing muscle strain. It is also an area that often narrows, showing a lack of strength in the structure of the midback caused by poor posture. The lower back is seen on the end of the nose. This area is a little harder to read because there are so many markings that indicate the functioning of the heart. Look for changes in the quality of the flesh of the nose. For example, an indentation at the side of the tip would indicate a muscle weakness in the lower back. If this area is pinched, it shows a compression of the spine in the lower back.

All of these markings on the nose are very subtle, but in my practice and in the practices of the chiropractors and osteopaths who are my students, they have been very accurate diagnostic signs of back problems.

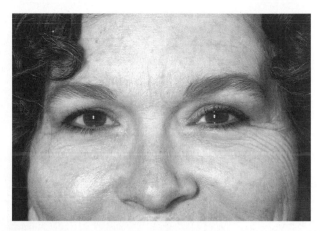

FIGURE 7-15.   The woman in this photo has very strong cheekbones, which is a sign of bossiness. In addition, she has a lot of pride and the ability to speak authoritatively.

CHEEKBONES AND UPPER CHEEKS

The cheekbones are like the shoulders of the face. My mother used to call them the hangers for the skin. She said that if you had cheekbones, it held your skin up better, and it kept you looking younger because your skin was less likely to sag. Large cheekbones (Figure 7-15) are correlated with strong metal energy. One of the traits of large cheekbones is pride. When people have a lot of pride, they take good care of themselves and therefore won't age as fast. Cheekbones also show bossiness. If you have noticeable cheekbones, you may be bossy. There are actually two parts to the cheekbones, the bark and the bite. The bark is the front part of the cheekbones under the eyes. Someone with this trait acts bossy but does not necessarily follow through with much authority. Cheekbones that are strong on the side below the temple reveal the bite. This implies consequences when demands are not carried through. Individuals with these cheekbones expect people to listen. This is a sign of great authority that carries an underlying threat of shunning if the recipient of this energy does not do what is expected. The difference between the two is the underlying power. People with front cheekbones want people to listen. People with side cheekbones expect it. And, if someone has both, this person has to be listened to!

Fleshy padding over the cheekbone incicates a person who bosses so nicely that you hardly notice that you are told what to do. The extra flesh makes this person friendlier. If the cheekbones are bony and angular, the bearer doesn't mince words when being bossy. Requests are made in a pointed way, and the words sound sharp. Cheekbones that are slanted downward from the temple area toward the mouth (Figure 7-16) are a sign of adventurousness. This kind of adventure usually involves travel to foreign lands or even the ability to be adventurous about food or entertainment choices.

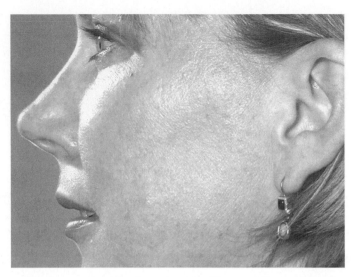

FIGURE 7-16. The woman in this photo has cheekbones with a strong diagonal line that indicates her need for adventure. This may include a desire to travel or to try new and different experiences.

Small cheekbones (Figure 7-17) reveal a person who doesn't like being bossed or being the boss. When the cheekbone area is flat, hollowed, or indented, the bearer has authority and self-esteem issues. These people do not like being told what to do and really dislike telling others what to do. They prefer to be left alone to work. They cannot stand having someone watching over them, and they are

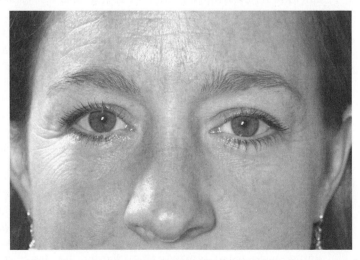

FIGURE 7-17. The woman in this photo has small cheekbones, which shows that she does not like being told what to do and doesn't really enjoy telling others what to do either. She believes in "live and let live" and needs to feel that she is self-directed.

usually not satisfied with what they accomplish. They often lack pride in their work. In fact, they usually think that anybody could have done what they did. They prefer not to give advice and are more likely to tell a story about what they did in a similar circumstance and hope that they are helping by example.

The cheek area is one of the most important areas for monitoring the health of the lungs. This area, called the "breath of life area," is directly below the cheekbones and above the jaw area. It borders and crosses into the moneybags area that belongs to the earth element. The cheeks show the current functioning of the lungs. Any sign of indentation, hollowing, or discoloration indicates a problem with the lungs. This area is the first to show stress, which inhibits proper lung functioning. Living life in a hurry, excessive stress, breathing shallowly, not living in the present, or feeling chronic lack and deprivation all contribute to lung deficiency. Healthy lungs are shown here by firm skin that is neither too tight nor too loose and by a faint pink color, which is a sign of proper oxygenation of the body.

THE SPACES ON THE FACE

When someone has strength in the metal element, this person values order and cleanliness. There is a strong need for space and a dislike of being closed in. Metallic people cultivate serenity and have naturally refined faces. They also exhibit a lot of space between the features; this is the air aspect of the element. Because metal is symbolized by the color white, these spaces can also be called "white spaces" on the face. These include the space across the forehead, the distance between the eyebrows and eyes, the length between the nose and mouth, and the width between the cheekbones. The metal element embodies reflection and detachment, and so do these spaces.

A wide distance across the forehead indicates open-mindedness and a philosophical bent. Width between the eyebrows is a sign of tolerance, acceptance, and a lack of judgment. Widely spaced eyes belong to people who have breadth of vision and see the big picture. Close-set eyes show an attention to detail. Both are signs of metal. Cheekbones that are far apart indicate a person who has the ability to be a leader. A narrower space between cheekbones is a sign of a loner, which is also a metal aspect.

A longer length in the philtrum area (the groove between the nose and mouth) indicates a person who can take teasing because it isn't taken that personally (Figure 7-18). They are removed from any feeling of attack and can enjoy practical jokes. When this area is short (Figure 7-19), this person is very touchy and sensitive and cannot take that kind of humor because it penetrates and hurts. Both are signs of metal. The amount of eyelid showing is also correlated to the metal element. Deep, hollow upper eyelids are metallic because they show grief and suffering from previous love relationships.

The amount of eyelid that covers the iris of the eye is another metal-based trait. If the eyelid covers up part of the iris, the bearer is a private person.

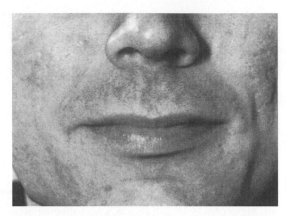

FIGURE 7-18.   The length of the philtrum on this man's face shows that he is capable of being the focus of teasing and joking. He doesn't take it personally.

When the eyelid droops in the center, creating a straight line across the iris, the bearer is a very fair and objective person (Figure 7-20). This person can see another's point of view. This shows strength in the metal element. When the eyelid comes down over the outside corners (Figure 7-21) the bearer has been criticized in the past and is self-critical. The right side shows criticism from the mother, wife, or other important female figure, and the left side shows criticism from father, husband, or other important male figure. This is a sign of metal deficiency because criticism acts like pinpricks to the balloon of the lungs. It is also highly correlated to autoimmune diseases because, ultimately, criticism from without is internalized and becomes self-criticism that attacks the self. Eyelids that droop on the inside and outside of the eye create what is called the "triangle eye." This is a trait that correlates to abuse in the past. People with this trait have shut down their emotions, especially kindness and compassion. This is a sign of severe metal deficiency and ego problems. Resentment and blame are used to cover up a deep sense of inadequacy, and hatred is a common emotion.

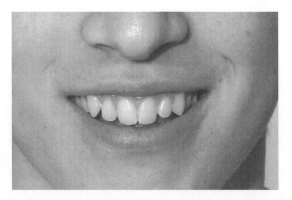

FIGURE 7-19.   The short area of the philtrum on this young man's face shows how sensitive he is to teasing and to jokes about him. He is touchy and takes things personally.

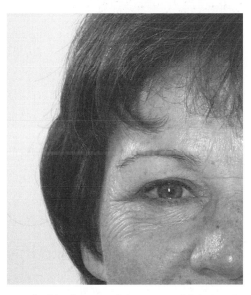

FIGURE 7-20.   The woman in this photograph has an eyelid that covers up the iris in a straight line. This shows that she is an objective person who can see both sides of a situation. She is not judgmental and is very fair in her actions.

The distance between the eyebrows and eyes is another sign of metal energy. Eyebrows that are set high above the eyelids are a sign of strong pride and high personal expectations. This is seen as eyebrows that are above the brow bone (Figure 7-22). People with this trait appear aloof and distant. They often believe that they know best. Their boundaries are strong, and they do not let anyone in unless they have feelings of trust. This trait can be manufactured by holding the

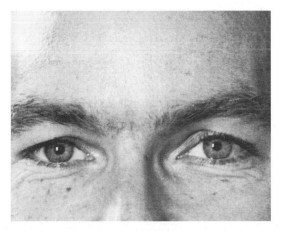

FIGURE 7-21.   The man in this photo has eyelids that come down across the outsides of his eyes. This indicates that he has either been criticized in the past or is self-critical. However, it has also made his standards higher and his thinking more precise.

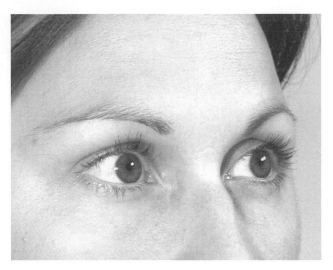

FIGURE 7-22.   The woman in this photo has eyebrows that are above the brow bone and are also relatively high. This makes her appear slightly aloof but is actually a sign of enhanced pride.

eyebrows higher in a look of surprise or skepticism, or the eyebrow hairs can be tweezed to make the eyebrows look farther away. In either case, the distance created intensifies the metal trait and can even be called *metal excess.*

The opposite occurs when people have eyebrows close to their eyelids (Figure 7-23). These are called "coach's eyebrows." They belong to friendly, affable people who have high expectations for other people (not necessarily for themselves) and

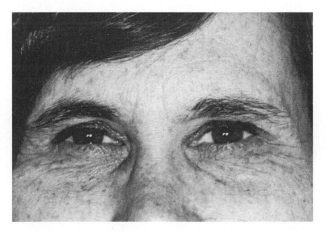

FIGURE 7-23.   The woman in this photo has eyebrows close to her eyes and shows that she is friendly. She gets very involved with the people she works with or cares about and tries to mentor them.

get very personally involved with people whom they are trying to mold and change. For example, I once knew a great track coach who hated to run but made a lot of young men into track stars by training them.

The lower the eyebrows, the more involved these people get with their protégés. There are few, if any, boundaries with these eyebrows. The relationships that these people get into are very symbiotic and intensely personal. They have trouble separating themselves from those close to them. As mentors or parents, they look at their charges as ego extensions. If the mentees do well, the mentor has done a good job. Low eyebrows indicate a metal deficiency. Eyebrows that are high enough to show the eyes clearly, but not too high, signify balanced metal energy. This is a sign of self-confidence and healthy boundaries. Individuals with these eyebrows have a clear sense of self versus other.

SKIN

The skin is often called the third lung. It breathes by opening and closing the pores. It is the first line of resistance or defense against the environment. It is the easiest place to monitor current lung function. Problems with the complexion show that the lungs are weak and that other organs or emotions are dominating the lungs. The first thing to look for is coloration. With the skin, you look for the five basic colors of the different organ groups: black for the kidneys, green for the liver, red for the heart, yellow for the earth, and white for the lungs. These colors appear in the shadows of the face or as a faint underlay of the skin. If any of these colors predominate, the associated organ is dominating the body and overacting on the lungs. Black is also the color of stagnation, green the color of toxicity, red the color of inflammation, yellow the color of putrefaction, and white the color of frozen lungs.

Skin texture is also important. If the skin is very dry, it is a sign of dehydration. If the skin is very oily, the liver is most likely in distress, as it is unable to process fats properly. When the skin is very dark, it shows a deep-seated illness or depression the kidneys are probably very overworked. If the skin is very red, there is too much fire in the lungs and in the body. This means that outside irritants have invaded the natural boundaries of the skin or that someone or something has gotten under your skin. This includes welts, hives, and rashes. If the skin is too tight because of excess fat, there is too much earth energy in the body. This is a sign of spleen dampness, potential obesity, and (often) high blood pressure and diabetes. Skin that is very pale and lacks color is a sign of blood deficiency and a lack of energy.

Healthy lungs and deep breathing create a glow on the skin with a light pink color, indicating proper oxygenation of the skin. The color of the skin also has a connection to the heart because the lungs and heart work so closely together. The emotion of grief from the lungs ravages the face more than any other. The emotion of love from the heart makes the face beautiful. Because the lungs are so tied to the functioning of the immune system, the skin is one of the best places to begin to monitor health. That leads us into analyzing even more specific signs of facial diagnosis.

PART III

The Universal Language of the Face

"When the eyes say one thing, and the tongue another, a practiced man relies on the language of the first."
RALPH WALDO EMERSON, *THE CONDUCT OF LIFE*

The face has a language all its own. Once you learn to translate the signs on the face, you have gained access to the personality, inner emotions, and health of just about anyone. We have been scrutinizing the faces of others since we were born and attempting to interpret the expressions that we see. Yet we are not as good at receiving and processing this emotional information as we could be because we don't trust what we perceive. The information received from facial expressions is actually much more specific than words or gestures. However, the most accurate assessment of emotions comes from reading the changes in the light of the eyes that the ancient Chinese called the *shen*.

Shen is the spirit emanating from the eyes. It is a quality of light that glows from within that changes moment to moment. The *shen* shifts with different mood states and feelings. Body language can be controlled or manipulated, and the face can be forced into expressions that are not felt, but the *shen* never lies. It is the manifestation of the autonomic nervous system, which is not under voluntary control. In effect, when you learn to read the changes in the *shen*, you are becoming a living lie detector. An actual lie detector machine is called a *galvanic skin response meter*. This equipment operates by detecting changes in the activity of the nervous system or body processes, such as the amount of perspiration, through electrodes placed on the tips of the finger that monitor the rate of activity on a machine that graphs the changes. However, the human body is even better than a machine at picking up emotional information from another person. We usually feel and react to emotions without even having to process them mentally.

The ancient Chinese focused on five basic emotions: fear, anger, joy, worry, and grief. Each emotion is manifested differently through the *shen*. Learning to read other people's feelings and emotions by monitoring changes in the *shen* is an invaluable tool in interpersonal communication. It builds understanding and empathy. As stated by Daniel Goleman in *Emotional Intelligence*, "The benefits of being able to read feelings from non-verbal cues includes being better adjusted emotionally, more popular, more outgoing, and—perhaps not surprisingly—more sensitive."[1] In other words, learning to read expressions gives you a very high emotional IQ.

The ability to detect lying is one of the most useful tools in interpersonal communication, but most people don't do it very well. Dr. Paul Ekman, in his book, *Telling Lies: Clues to Deceit in the Marketplace, Marriage and Politics*, estimates that the majority of the population cannot tell whether they are being deceived and that Secret Service men are the best at pinpointing a lie because they are so observant and watch people.[2] They were accurate about 75% of the time, on average.[3] Psychologist Bella DePaula, of the University of Virginia, reported that she found that people lied 77% of the time with strangers, 48% with acquaintances, and 28% with good friends.[4] Most people lied to look smarter or kinder or in some way compliment themselves or protect someone else. Wouldn't it be helpful to be able to detect lies even a little better? Learning to read the subtle changes in the *shen* can help in this. Lying disturbs the *shen* by shutting down and hardening the heart. It limits the amount of emotion that can be expressed and creates a flat affect.

Carl Jung once stated, "Emotions are contagious." His conclusion has been backed up by current studies from Dr. Elaine Hatfield of the University of Hawaii. She likens emotions to social viruses, with some people having a natural ability to transmit them and other people being more likely to receive them. Moods are transmitted and returned within milliseconds—even unconsciously. Many other studies show that the pupils dilate in response to positive stimulus or things that interest people and that other people are attracted to this dilation. The wider the pupils dilate, the more the *shen* can show. It is actually easier to see the eyes get brighter or dimmer than to figure out whether the pupils are dilating or contracting. Some people have naturally larger pupils and brighter *shen*, but everyone can express *shen* naturally or deliberately to attract others. This vibratory expressiveness is called "peach luck." The Chinese used the peach to represent sex appeal and immortality.

Peach luck is a magical emanation that can also be called charisma, charm, or sex appeal. This is a personal and concentrated form of the fire energy directed outward to attract others, consciously or unconsciously. Everyone has some peach luck, and there are several different kinds. People can have the same kind of peach

[1]Goleman D: *Emotional Intelligence*, New York, Bantam Books, 1997.
[2]Ekman P: *Telling Lies: Clues to Deceit in the Marketplace, Marriage and Politics*, 2nd ed., New York, WW Norton, 2001.
[3]Maugh TH: The truth about lies: most honestly can't detect them, *Los Angeles Times*, Sep 5, 1991.
[4]Hawkes N: Truth to tell, liars are not easy to spot, *London Times*, Sep 8, 1997.

luck in varying degrees, or they can have and convey all five types. Peach luck is a necessary quality for people in professions such as the performing arts, politics, and evangelism. It is certainly also helpful in the everyday world for finding a mate or selling a product. Peach luck is something that starts off as innate and then can be developed. Learn what type of peach luck you are most attracted to and which kind you transmit.

The ability to read the face for clues about the health is *facial diagnosis*. Pathological conditions in the body can be seen on special areas of the face that correspond to each organ (as outlined in the previous chapters). This is like reading a biological blueprint. Diagnosing from the face involves evaluating the overuse or underuse of any organ's energy. These conditions of strength and weakness can be clearly seen in the facial features that correspond to each organ. The color of the area and the particular markings all give valuable clues about the body's function. The ancient Chinese did not actually diagnose diseases; instead, they treated symptoms. They believed that two people with malaria needed different treatments based on their particular needs. Therefore they looked to the face to diagnose the symptoms of excess or deficiency, inflammation, stagnation, coldness, dampness, or heat.

Five-element personality types associated with the different symptoms and syndromes can also be seen on the face; so can the psychological and emotional issues that contribute to a disease state. The face reveals so many clues about health that are there just waiting to be deciphered. Many of the diseases that are the leading causes of death have signs that appear on the face long before the disease becomes deadly. You cannot learn to look at someone and determine that the person has a certain disease, but you can learn to see predispositions and potential outcomes, all of which can be worked with to change the course of someone's illness or to enhance health.

There are gifts and lessons from every syndrome, disability, and disease. Sometimes it is important to be sick. The ancient Chinese had a marvelous saying, "Bless every illness because it has not yet killed you." They believed illness taught you the right way to go from that point on, to correct you so you could steer yourself away from the dangerous direction that you were headed. Facial diagnosis shows how the biological blueprint of your body's function is written in code on your face and then, in turn, deciphers that code.

8 / *Signs from the Shen*

"*Shen* is something that you will recognize when you see it. The *shen* can be observed through the patient's eyes."
THE YELLOW EMPEROR'S CLASSIC OF ORIENTAL MEDICINE[1]

The *shen* creates the look in the eyes that makes them appear backlit (Color Plate 13). This glow alters subtly in response to changes in moods and can be read moment to moment. All of the emotions can be seen in the eyes, and each emotion changes the quality of the *shen*. The ancient Chinese considered five emotions to be the most important. These five emotions were called the rebels of the body and needed to kept under control: fear from the kidneys, anger from the liver, joy or excitement from the heart, worry from the spleen/stomach, and sorrow or grief from the lungs. These emotions are a necessary part of the human experience and have value when used in balance. However, both overuse and underuse of these basic emotions can cause harm to the organ to which they belong. None of these emotions are bad emotions. It is a problem when you do not manage the expression of them or you suppress the release of them. Each of these major emotions also affects the face in specific ways and can be seen from the large amount or lack of markings on the face.

In the *Nei Jing, The Yellow Emperor's Classic of Oriental Medicine*, it is stated that, "When one is angry, the *ch'i* rises upward; when one is joyous, the *ch'i* disperses; when one is sad, the *ch'i* becomes exhausted; when one is fearful and frightened, the *ch'i* descends; when one is chilled, the *ch'i* contracts; when one is hot, the *ch'i* escapes; when one is anxious (excited), the *ch'i* scatters and becomes chaotic; when one overstrains, the *ch'i* depletes; when one worries too much, the *ch'i* stagnates." Feeling, expressing, or repressing these emotions all have effects on the body and eventually show on the face.

---

[1]Ni M: *The Yellow Emperor's Classic of Oriental Medicine*, Boston, Shambhala, 1995.

FEAR

Fear is the most primal of all the emotions and the one we arrive with from the trauma of our birth experience. We spend the rest of our lives trying to deal with and conquer our myriad fears. It is an ongoing battle for most people to fight their fear. Fear arises with most new and different circumstances and at times when a current situation resembles a time from the past when we were hurt or harmed. Fear is also common when people imagine future scenarios of loss or pain. When an individual feels afraid, the energy in the body drops down to protect the vital organs. The sphincter muscles, which are controlled by the kidneys, want to loosen to release any stored bodily fluids or solids. In this fight-or-flight mode, the body attempts to eliminate any unnecessary function to prepare for attack or to flee. This is why people feel tremendous pressure to relieve themselves when terrified. This is one of the fundamental responses to danger, real or imagined.

Fear first shows up in the eyes as a startle response. The eyes snap open, and then the *qi* freezes. Someone in this stage of fear looks much like a deer caught in the headlights. This look of shock is often accompanied by raised eyebrows. Then there is the reaction of pulling backward, often literally but primarily with the energy. The *qi* drops downward, and the light is lost from the eyes. The eyes end up looking darker and murkier. This is the sign of dread.

Overuse of fear depletes the kidneys. This is seen on the face as dark circles and hollowness under the eyes. It also exhausts the adrenals, and this is seen as red-rimmed lower eyelids, or three-white-sided eyes when severe. If chronic, it can show up as a weakening in the structure of the chin (in the fleshy area) and makes the chin look like an orange peel. This kind of chin appears wobbly, and the flesh does not appear to be well attached to the bone. This is an indication of a lack of will and courage caused by deficient kidneys. People who have been in chronic fear hold their eyes open too wide and appear to be in a constant state of shock. The darkness in their eyes is a sign of frozen *qi* and inability to move through the fear they are holding within. Fear is slow to debilitate but, when held for long periods, weakens the *jing* and causes premature aging. Therefore any signs of premature aging are signs of overuse of the kidneys, overuse of the will, or chronic fear.

Fear can be a valuable emotion when felt in moderation. It creates caution and an early warning system that helps protect us from potential harm. When real and not imaginary, it galvanizes the body into preparation for fight or flight.

ANGER

Anger is a very powerful emotion that is used as both a shield for defense and a weapon. It is probably the most expressed and validated emotion in the Western world. Anger destroys and also creates change. The ancient Chinese described anger as the *qi* rising upward, making your face flush and your eyes bulge. Anger is also a very focused emotion and creates hardness and tightness in the body in preparation for fighting and attack. If anger is a constant emotion, it causes hardening of the body, leading to rigid thinking and problems with adaptation and change.

It is easiest to see anger in the narrowing of the eyes and mouth, the flaring of the nostrils, the lowering of the eyebrows, and the furrows that are created between the eyebrows. The face in anger is hard, and the *shen* becomes concentrated and intense. Anger is an energetic attack that affects the recipient in a specific place in his or her body. Everyone reacts to anger differently. For some, it attacks the stomach, others, the heart or head. Anger is so strong that it can attack you even if it is not directed at you. You can just be around an angry person and absorb it. Later, when you have a tight chest or an upset stomach, you might want to think back to some anger you absorbed through your most vulnerable organ. Anger is so pervasive in our society that it is almost an epidemic.

When overused, anger is seen as very deep lines between the eyebrows, and the whole area has a reddish cast. The sclera (white part of the eyes) is chronically red, the face has hardened into a mask, the lips are held very tight, and the jaw is clenched. Eventually, the jaw structure will weaken, the eyebrows will lose hair, the area between the eyebrows will become sunken and hollow under the wrinkles, and the sclera will darken and have a yellow-green-gray appearance. These are signs of overuse or toxicity of the liver. They can be caused by other sources besides anger. Certainly the liver enjoys processing toxins, but too much anger is very toxic, especially when it is in the form of hate. It festers and poisons the person who feels it.

Correct use of anger is a valuable tool. It is a powerful weapon and a protective shield against abuse. It creates change, not in a precise way but through massive destruction of the old. It is the foundation of power. However, one must guard against the hardening of the tree, because it becomes more susceptible to falling in the wind. Flexibility is an asset, and anger is best used only when truly needed.

JOY OR EXCITEMENT

The ancient Chinese had a great fear of excess fire. They cautioned repeatedly in their writings and teachings to beware of burning up your *qi*. They warned not to get too excited or too sad; they believed in moderation of all the emotions and especially of the fire element, which was translated as joy. I believe that this was and is a mistranslation. I think they really meant that excess excitement—mania—was damaging to the heart. Joy, which is defined by *Webster's Dictionary* as "a very glad feeling; happiness; great pleasure" is surely not dangerous. However, living off your adrenaline and constantly seeking higher levels of excitement and sensory experiences is exhausting and ultimately harmful to the body. Excitement causes your energy to become scattered and chaotic. It is a very attractive emotion. The eyes widen and brighten, the *shen* flares, the mouth opens slightly, and the nervous system begins to vibrate at a very high frequency. Excitement is fun in the short term and exhausting in the long term. It is an emotion that is much too commonly sought out in the Western world. There are large numbers of adrenaline junkies and sensation seekers who constantly strive for bigger and better thrills. Peaceful, calm living is seen as boring and soul-killing.

In reality, the soul can't emerge if the body is operating too quickly. Living on an emotional roller coaster is another life style that overuses the fire energy. Frequently expressing all feelings on a grand scale leaves little time for contemplation, rest, or deep feeling. It is hard to recover from the exhaustion that comes from living with emotional extremes, and those who are used to living this way collapse, only to build up just enough energy to do it again. Excitement is temporary and fleeting.

After a period of intense excitement comes the letdown and the other fire emotion—sadness. Although many books on Chinese medicine categorize this emotion as part of the lung energies, I see it as the aftereffect of too much excitement and emotion. It is the dropping heart and the corollary letdown of the *shen*. The heart is tired. Sadness is part of the rebound effect that leads to the quest for more excitement instead of peace. When the sadness leads to tears, it becomes sorrow and then grief, both of which are lung emotions. It is important to note how closely connected the heart and lungs are, as is shown in medicine, where the heart and lung are considered to be functioning as part of the cardiopulmonary system.

The signs of excess fire are chronic redness in the neck, throat, and face. This is redness that is constant, not temporary. Diseases involving inflammation are also an indication of excess fire energy, as are problems with speech and thinking. False fire is another condition of which to be wary. False fire looks very similar to excess fire but has no real energy to support the action. There is also not enough real fire to put the fire out—or to put the false fire out until exhaustion finally does the job. False fire occurs when individuals attempts to act vivacious, cheerful, talkative, or happy when they are not. This is a form of acting that is much validated by our society. We appreciate people acting happy, but this can exhaust the heart if the emotions expressed are not real.

Living dramatically with a life style that is too scattered, mobile, changeable, and unstable can wear out the heart. Using too much emotion is also exhausting. The resulting burnout is often first seen as a lack of emotional energy or a lack of affect—the inability to feel anything. This eventually leads to immobility, a lack of physical energy to do anything. A severe lack of fire can be seen in an inappropriately pale complexion, a dullness of the *shen*, and a heavily downturned mouth. Other signs are the inability to handle new and different stimuli or being easily overstimulated and overwhelmed. This can also lead to false fire, often diagnosed as attention deficit hyperactivity disorder or other neurological problems. There is not enough fire to fight fire. Rest is certainly called for, although for people who enjoy living on the fire energy, rest is considered boring. In addition, once rested, they simply get up and burn up their fire energy again. It is much better to build up the fire energy for when you really want to use it. Simple living, subtle pleasures, emotions kept under control, and just enough stimulation to stave off boredom are all ways to rebuild the fire energy.

WORRY AND CONFUSION

The earth element is represented in the body by the spleen and stomach. The emotion involved with these organs is worry. The worrying usually involves someone else, as people with a lot of earth energy are very other-directed. Worry has no resolution; it is a repetitive process that is like a hamster on an exercise wheel. The ancient Chinese believed that it led to stagnation. You never really get anywhere when you worry except back to where you started. Worry leads to confusion as the thinking becomes involved. The thinking is repetitive and obsessive and is accompanied by a churning feeling in the gut. Worry is an attempt to stay connected with people you care about, even when they are not present. This is a very maternal or paternal energy. There is rarely an attempt to do anything about the worry, but the act of worrying itself makes it feel as though you are doing something for someone that you love.

Worry causes the *qi* to stagnate. The energy gets stuck in the brain and in the stomach, resulting in unclear thinking and incomplete digestion. It is believed to contribute to weight gain. The eyes appear to have a lost look. They often appear glazed and unfocused. If you look very carefully at the *shen,* you see that the light of the eye vibrates, and sometimes even the eyeball itself moves slightly in a back-and-forth or circular fashion. This is the sign of frantic thought behind what appears to be a calm surface.

Worry never solves anything. The feelings are never released but, instead, are held onto and replayed over and over again. Repetitive thinking and action result in stagnation that can turn into a quagmire. It keeps people "stomping in the swamp," dealing with unresolved feelings and muddied thoughts instead of being able to move on. It creates indecisiveness and the need to find authority outside the self. It can lead to someone becoming a "lost soul." The soul's intent is buried beneath whirling thoughts and recycled feelings. This stagnation caused by excess earth also affects the body and creates many problems of absorption and digestion. It affects the fluidity of the sticky body fluids such as saliva, lymph fluid, and blood and can cause circulation problems and clotting. There may be excessive weight gain that can be seen around the middle of the body and in the upper arms and lower calves. It can lead to emotional eating and overeating. There may be compression of the body, with such problems as fallen arches or compressed vertebrae and problems of containment such as hemorrhoids or edema (water retention). There is often a puffy look on the face, especially in the lips, eyelids, and lower cheeks.

When the earth element has been overused, it leads to earth deficiency. This is revealed in the inability to absorb and retain. It can impact memory, as the mind has trouble absorbing new ideas or remembering. Earth deficiency in the body shows up as the inability to digest food, like the inability to digest sugar in diabetes, or the inability to take in food or keep the food, as in anorexia and bulimia. This would also show on the face as an inability to gain weight, and hollowness in the cheeks or having a body with very little body fat are signs of earth deficiency.

There is an up side to worry and the resulting confusion that it causes. The usefulness of worry is that it can help delay decisions and helps prevent impulsiveness. When parents worry about their children or friends worry about each other, worry becomes attached to love, and many people would not feel loved if their parents or spouse weren't worrying about them. It is a familial way of staying connected and attached.

GRIEF

The last basic emotion of the five elements is the metal emotion of grief. This emotion is felt the deepest and may compromise the immune system the most. Grief is not something that we in the Western world are allowed to express much. In fact, in the United States it is considered unseemly to show too much grief, even at a funeral. We admire people who hold their emotions in and keep themselves controlled and composed. People are allowed to show and share their grief for approximately 3 months following a loss. After that, they need to internalize it and are given up to 1 year to process their loss as if that was all the time necessary to get over it. One of the latest phrases about grief that is in common usage is, "needing to get closure." This shows the belief that grief is supposed to have an ending.

In other parts of the world, it is considered proper to show extreme grief, to prostrate oneself in front of the coffin, weep profusely, or wail uncontrollably. This gets the emotions out. Widows are allowed to wear their mourning clothes for as long as they want, sometimes for the rest of their lives. In a completely opposite way, some cultures encourage celebrations of someone's life, as in the Irish wakes or the Balinese parades. They are attempting to find goodness in tragedy, and they combine laughter with the pain of loss.

Grief shows in the eyes as a deadness of the *shen*, which feels heavy to the observer. The eyes do not sparkle. Even if people who are grieving smile with their mouths, their eyes won't reciprocate. The lack of *shen* in the eyes can be confused with the dullness of depression or the murkiness of fear, but the corollary signs, hollowing and darkening of the cheeks and an overall ashen or gray color of the skin, attest to the emotion of grief at the core. The deadness of the *shen* is deeper, and there is no anger simmering below or fear behind it. Instead, there is tiredness because grief has no end. Grief doesn't just stop; it only lessens in severity over time. I do not believe that you really ever get over losing someone that you love. You just get better at dealing with the loss and going on with your life.

Grief can be an overwhelming emotion and has been shown to lower the immune function faster than any other emotion. The ancient Chinese doctors believed that grief causes the *qi* to become exhausted. It diminishes the capacity of the lungs to take air in and compromises the ability to breathe out the toxins. Grief limits life and the ability to live with any zest. I believe that the spirit of the person left behind tries to go with the spirit that has left, and this does not leave enough spirit in the body to live fully, only partially. Therefore it is important to take the time necessary to process grief but avoid trying to hold onto those who have left you.

You need to stay here, in the present, and continue your life. The metal element is about the future.

SHEN DISTURBANCE: READING LIES, TELLING TRUTH

The truth is a valuable thing, especially when given with compassion. Truth can be seen as clarity of light in the eye. People with clear *shen* are true to themselves and others. However, because truth is often used as a weapon, most people in society lie in various ways to protect themselves, the feelings of others, or their egos.

Lying changes the quality of shen. It shuts down and hardens the heart and lowers the amount of light emanating from the eyes. If done frequently and repeatedly, it can lead to an inability to feel compassion and eyes that appear dull or dead. Many drugs, such as tranquilizers, can lead to a similar look, as can severe depression. However, most people tell the truth or at least part of the truth most of the time. How do you detect lying?

The first thing to look for is whether someone looks at you when speaking. Most people look away when they are lying. That makes it hard to see the *shen*. However, the very act of looking away is a clue. This action has a furtive quality about it caused by the fear of being discovered. Because fear is from water and the *shen* is from fire, the fear of getting caught causes the *shen* to shut down, and the eye's light dims or temporarily disappears (water overacts on fire). It must be noted that some people look away because they are very shy or their culture does not permit staring. This should not be considered a sign of lying.

Although most people will tell you that they don't tell lies, in actuality, most people lie every day. These lies are often excused as "white lies" or lies by omission. Part of the truth is told, but not all. These kinds of lies are considered harmless and help lubricate social interaction. They are actually considered socially acceptable. The white lie alters the *shen* just a little and only for a fraction of a second because, although part of the conversation is a lie, the rest of it is truth. The lessening of light in the eyes is very subtle, like a camera shutter closing.

However, even very good liars have changes that occur in the *shen*. Good liars have less fear, so they can look right at you and act very sincere, usually overly sincere.

Chronic liars also exaggerate. There is usually a lot of charm involved. These kinds of people lie for maximal effect. They are performers who love pretending and are usually very quick thinking and very humorous. They continuously seek new audiences to impress. Their personalities are narcissistic, and they will do anything to make themselves look good, including lying. Underneath it all is a deep-seated insecurity. The *shen* in this case is very bright but very cool. There is no real warmth or empathy that can be felt from their expression.

The ancient Chinese labeled severe liars as criminals. Even before they ever committed a crime, they were viewed with great suspicion. If the *shen* was too bright and there was not enough of the earth element or the signs of morality on the face, these people would never be put in positions of power over money or other people because they would take advantage of them. Today, we call people who function

through lies sociopaths. Sociopaths enjoy gullible people and can be found bla-
tantly telling falsehoods. Lying is like a game to them, and so is life. They are not
usually bothered by being caught lying. In fact, they tend to admire those who are
smart enough to see through their lies. They can shut off their feelings easily and
prefer living in the realm of the facile mind. These people believe that they are
mentally superior, and if people are too stupid to see through their lies, then they
deserve to be lied to. Their minds are very quick, and they must have a good
memory to remember all the lies they have told. There is an air of arrogance and a
steely quality to their eyes. They smile with their mouths but not their eyes. The *shen*
in a sociopath is glittery and cold. They can be glib talkers but exude no warmth in
their *shen* or in their actions.

Psychopaths lack *shen* altogether. Their eyes are like deep wells of darkness. It is
not like the dullness caused by depression or the murkiness of emotional distress.
It is much heavier. When looking into a psychopath's eyes, you feel the chill of
death. It is such a strong trait that it can even be seen in photographs. Psychopaths
are driven by their need to victimize others, like psychic vampires living off other
people's energy. They are attracted energetically to those whose *shen* is temporarily
fragile. Their own lack of *shen* could be described as anti-*shen*. They project a
perverse sort of magnetism that can suck others in but usually remains hidden until
someone is chosen as a victim. The energy is repulsive, yet fascinating. It is the dark
and scary underworld of *shen* at its most *yin* point, going down to the place where
there is no *shen* to be seen.

However, as in all things in the world, there must be an opposite for psycho-
pathic *shen*, and there is. The lightest and most *yang* point of *shen* is also the most
positive aspect of *shen* projection, the magical and mesmerizing qualities of peach
luck. This is when the *shen* is emanated at the highest vibration to attract others in
a positive way. Peach luck is the embodiment of light that attracts others like moths
fluttering toward a flame.

THE POWER OF PEACH LUCK

There is another language of the face that is the language of attraction. What makes
people attractive to others? Why are some people so charismatic and magnetic?
Some people always seem to attract others to them easily and naturally. Is it because
of good looks? Is it a certain smile? Having a great personality? What these people
have a lot of and everybody has some of is the ancient Chinese peach luck. Peach
luck is a name for charisma, charm, and sex appeal.

Peach luck is that special quality expressed primarily in the eyes that magnetizes
others to you. It is the sexual energy expressed through the *shen* but is refined so
that it can be expressed in public. Peach luck was originally called "peach blossom
luck" because of the beauty of the flowers when they bloomed in spring and was
compared to the flowery, flirtatious look in the eyes. Eventually the peach itself was
also seen as enticing. The beautiful colors, seductive aroma, soft skin, and luscious
flesh all invite you to take a bite. That's why the Chinese used the peach as a symbol
of sex appeal and immortality. Interestingly, some theologians have hypothesized

that the apple from the Garden of Eden might actually have been a peach. That makes more sense to me. If you're going to be tempted, peaches are definitely more sensual than apples.

A high degree of peach luck is necessary for people involved in charismatic professions such as sales, politics, the ministry, and entertainment. People in these professions rely on their popularity, which comes from their ability to influence and attract many people to them. It also accounts for the great fame some people maintain even after their death. When people die at the height of their peach luck, they are immortalized. They are said to have died in full bloom.

People with peach luck possess magnetism and have a special dynamism. Peach luck is comparable to the Pied Piper's music or Lorelei's song. People who are attracted to this energy do not always understand why, but they are drawn in nonetheless. It's why people swoon over certain movie or rock stars.

Peach luck is magical and mesmerizing. It casts a spell and draws you in, but it also has a dark side. It can be so compelling that it allows people to ignore otherwise questionable personality traits or behaviors and is one of the explanations for the lemminglike following of such dangerous leaders as Adolph Hitler and Jim Jones. In milder cases of deception or deceit, we forgive the sins of those with peach luck much more readily because these people are so charming even when they are wrong.

Some people have lots of peach luck, whereas others have very little. Luckily, everybody has some. You do not have to be beautiful to have peach luck. In fact, peach luck gives the illusion of beauty. It is an energy that emanates from the eyes that makes you look alive and appear fascinating. It is a show of your spirit manifested through the *shen* having been filtered through the five elements of experience.

When I first started learning about peach luck, I was taught lessons about how wonderful and terrible it was. I assumed that either you had it or you didn't, and luckily I was told I had some. I was also warned repeatedly to watch out for it because I was going to attract more attention than was good for me. My uncle used to tell me that I had so much that I could choose to have lots of men or to become famous. To me, choosing lots of men was a waste of this precious energy, whereas being famous could mean having a lonelier life. Peach luck actually scared me, and I tried to minimize it.

What I came to realize over time is that peach luck can be controlled, and it can also be cultivated. It is not a predestined energy. It involves opening your heart and being willing to show and share your spirit. I realized that babies are all born with peach blossom luck as they flirt and charm with their eyes and their smiles of delight. They are showing their excitement about being alive. Over time, this original joy can be nourished or suppressed. People who keep this original fire energetic and alive have the primary form of peach luck called sparkling peach luck. However, many people have traumatic lives, and their fire gets suppressed, as does their peach blossom luck. It still emerges, but in an altered form based on how much suffering has occurred. Although these other manifestations of peach luck are still intriguing and attracting, they are emitted through the filters of the elemental emotions.

Peach luck can therefore be divided into five types: sparkling, supportive, dreamy, seductive, and direct. Sparkling is most true to the original description of peach blossom luck and shows a heart that is most open to excitement and joy. The other four types show the defenses and shields that have been thrown up as protection for the heart, which changes the emission of joy as it is revealed to the world. Ultimately, the other forms of peach luck form a five-element cycle of emotional expression that, when completed, can bring people back to their true selves through the discovery of what makes them truly happy (Table 8-1).

SPARKLING PEACH LUCK

Sparkling peach luck is pure fire energy at its brightest. People who have this kind of peach luck are seen as fun, comical, charming, and delightful. They are just so cute! They laugh and smile easily, their eyes are bright, and their smiles are huge. They are said to "light up the room." Their smiles captivate. These people are playful, enthusiastic, and often mischievous. As with Peter Pan, this is the contagious charm of a child who never fully grew up. People with sparkling peach luck can stay out of trouble and get away with a lot just by laughing, smiling, or joking their way out of difficult situations.

This is the most popular type of peach luck in the entertainment industry. Comedic actors with this type of peach luck lift our spirits and make us feel better. They don't take life too seriously and don't want you to either. People with sparkling peach luck believe in having a good time, and they are here to show you how to enjoy life, too. They love champagne celebrations or anything that includes bubbles. This kind of peach luck makes life more like a party.

Ronald Reagan has lots of this kind of peach luck. While he was president, his eyes smiled even when his mouth didn't. His nickname was fitting: "the Teflon president." He had so much charm that he didn't stay in trouble long. He would forget someone's name and apologize with a smile, and all would be well.

TABLE 8-1   Signs of Peach Luck

ELEMENT	Fire	Earth	Metal	Water	Wood
TYPE	Sparkling	Supportive	Dreamy	Seductive	Direct
ENERGETIC QUALITIES	Effervescent	Empathetic	Visionary	Deep	Intense
	Bubbly	Comforting	Inspirational	Mysterious	Projects power
	Fun	Caring	Sensitive	Has suffered	Determined
	Playful	Warm	Wistful	Listens well	Appears dangerous
	Mischievous	Parental	Idealistic	Secretive	Shows leadership
	Enthusiastic	Kind	Spiritual	Wise	Strong opinions
	Charm	Rescues	Refined	Sensual	Focused
FACIAL INDICATORS	Bright eyes	Kind eyes	Soft eyes	Deep eyes	Intense gaze
	Big smile	Sweet smile	Slight smile	Knowing smile	Doesn't smile

Bill Clinton luckily has a lot of this kind of peach luck too, but not quite enough to stay out of trouble. Many of our favorite movie stars have this type of peach luck— Meg Ryan, Robin Williams, Billy Crystal, and Julia Roberts, just to name a few.

Sparkling peach luck (Color Plate 14) belongs to people who have never lost their sense of wonder about the world. They have not forgotten what it is like to be a child. They maintain their youthfulness of spirit and appear younger than they are. They have buoyant spirits and an optimistic nature. Their charm comes from an ongoing excitement about being alive and an inner fire that cannot be quenched.

SUPPORTIVE PEACH LUCK

The next form of peach luck is emanated from people who have been saddened by their lives and do not believe that life is as much fun as it used to be for them. Yet they know that for others it can be, so they become the supportive people who help others have a good time.

This kind of peach luck is as cozy and cuddly as a stuffed animal. This is the earth element as seen through the eyes. These people are not as happy-go-lucky as those with sparkling peach luck because they are a little sadder, but people who exhibit supportive peach luck are warm and caring. They are very maternal or paternal. They are always ready to give a hug and lots of sympathy. They are wonderful caretakers and give easily. Their eyes show their kindness and understanding, and they have a wonderfully sweet smile. They look as though they are always ready to feed you tea and cookies when times are good or bad because food makes everything seem better. They have great shoulders to cry on and give great comfort when times are bad. They are ready with the pep talk or encouragement when times are troubled. They really believe that everything will turn out all right.

This trait is very common for people in the helping professions. Look for plump cheeks and eyes with plenty of warmth. It is also a very common form of peach luck in talk show hosts. Think of Oprah Winfrey and her warmth and caring for her guests. This is the ideal type of peach luck in grandparents and caretakers. With supportive peach luck, there is an aura of approachability and softness and the promise of affection (Color Plate 15).

DREAMY PEACH LUCK

Dreamy peach luck is seen as a far-off gaze and eyes that are full of hope. Individuals with dreamy peach luck have suffered but still believe that life can be different than it is. If they just tried harder, they could make it so, someday. This type of peach luck is representative of the metal energy that is looking forward to the future because the present is just not up to their standards. They are disappointed in the reality of now and know and believe that it can be better.

Dreamy peach luck is an inspiring energy that touches the hopes and dreams of others and gives them some belief that ideals can come true. This look is often accompanied by a slightly wistful smile. People with this kind of peach luck are sensitive daydreamers. They have great imaginations and can be considered visionary and idealistic. They are not happy about life as it is, so they fantasize about making it better someplace, somewhere, some other time. They believe in utopia. They know that the world is far from perfect, but they believe it can be made to become more as it should be. The inspiration and beauty of their dreams can draw you in and make you believe that it is possible.

One of the best examples of a world leader who had dream peach luck is Martin Luther King, Jr. In almost all photos of him or film clips of his speeches, he has a faraway look in his eyes. His most famous speech is even entitled, "I Have a Dream." This extraordinary man was a visionary who drew people into his belief of a better world—someday. The shining light of his ideals is still a magnet to this day, many years after his death. That is the power of dreamy peach luck (Color Plate 16).

SEDUCTIVE PEACH LUCK

People with seductive peach luck look mysterious. They smile with a knowing smile, if they smile at all. They have a look of wisdom that is the water energy as seen through the eyes. Their eyes look watery and deep; they have been drawn farther into pain than most people but have come back with the knowledge of how to escape despair. By looking into their eyes, you can almost sense how bad it has been and how deeply they have suffered, but what you really want to know is how they have survived. This energy is called seductive because it draws other people out.

People who possess this form of peach luck are great listeners. People naturally volunteer very personal information to people with seductive peach luck. They know these people have knowledge to share. They can empathize with your pain and teach you how to survive the tragedies of life, but these people rarely reveal much about themselves. Their answers tend to be simplistic and yet powerfully true. They have experienced the drama of life and have gone beyond it. They look as if they can teach you how to cope. People with seductive peach luck have obviously suffered for love but are not afraid to keep on loving anyway. They give off a magnetism that promises passion and depth, intimacy, and awareness.

This is a very dramatic-looking form of peach luck (Color Plate 17) and can be seen on the faces of those who have suffered around the world. It can be seen in the faces of refugee children and their mothers, all of whom possess the haunting beauty of people who have experienced things beyond most people's imaginings. Seductive peach luck is beautiful because it is deep. Although the body and mind have suffered, the soul is still intact and shows through the eyes.

DIRECT PEACH LUCK

Direct peach luck is seen in the look that gets right to the point, wood energy at its maximal intensity. People with this kind of peach luck are able to focus their attention on their listeners and get their message across with no equivocation. The listener feels like either the only person in the room or a butterfly under a pin. The gaze of a person with direct peach luck probes and feels as though it goes right through you. People with direct peach luck project power and danger, both of which are considered potent aphrodisiacs. What's most unusual about this form of peach luck is that you don't have to like people who convey this energy, but you certainly can't ignore them. They can attract you even if you resist. They have an intense gaze and rarely smile. There is an edge to their magnetism that makes your heart beat faster and creates a feeling of helplessness. People with direct peach luck are natural leaders. They can compel you to follow, even if it is against your better judgment.

Many world leaders carry this aura of power and danger. It is obvious that crossing them is a mistake. These people have suffered to the point where they aren't going to take it anymore. They are going to have their way, and everyone in their path had better move out of the way. They are going to get what they want because they deserve it. They are driven and focused on the outcome. They believe that achieving will make them happy again.

Direct peach luck can be used by some of the most dangerous people in the world to control others and gain power and profit for their own benefit. We have seen direct peach luck used in evil ways, as in the case of Adolph Hitler and his powerful oratory. However, this form of peach luck is also much admired and desired in world leaders. The presidents and prime ministers of most countries have some of this form of peach luck. We want them to talk tough when necessary and show strong leadership abilities. The power they convey mesmerizes their constituency. In most cultures, talking tough is admired and respected. Direct peach luck (Color Plate 18) is very *yang* and is the force behind change for both good and bad. This form of peach luck involves conquest and victory, not negotiation.

DEVELOPING OR ENHANCING PEACH LUCK

All five types of peach luck are natural manifestations of the fire energy inherent in everyone's emotional makeup. How this fire energy is expressed depends on the willingness to express fire through the individual filter of each person's life experiences and on the individual's five element personality overlay. Societal pressures also influence the ability to express fire. For example, in China, children are cautioned against being too happy or showing too much sparkling peach luck. This energy is believed to lead to too much attraction from others and cause unstable marriages. In most cultures, direct peach luck is often valued in men but not in women. Because of this social conditioning, many people suppress their peach luck instead of expressing it.

Peach luck is the magical aspect of an individual's personality that is immortalized and remembered long after death. Charm is associated with sparkling peach luck, kindness with supportive peach luck, idealism with dreamy peach luck, mysteriousness with seductive peach luck, and power with direct peach luck.

Some people are capable of conveying a great deal of peach luck; others have only a little; but everyone has some. Most famous actors are capable of expressing at least two types of peach luck well. Others can express all five types of peach luck and have a chameleon–like quality that makes them appear to be different people in different situations. Peach luck is most powerful when used for the highest good.

People can pretend to have it or use what they have to manipulate others, but this isn't recommended. Peach luck is a projection of your spirit. Convey it with the best and clearest intent. When used with integrity, peach luck is pure magic. So how do you develop and enhance peach luck?

One of the best examples of a person who developed peach luck was Eleanor Roosevelt (Figure 8-1). She was a woman not naturally gifted with either beauty or charm. She was considered plain and shy. She did, however, possess wit, intelligence, and integrity that needed to be expressed. She ended up maturing to become a fascinating and magnetic public figure. Eleanor Roosevelt learned to accept herself despite what she considered her imperfections and became a happy person. She became known for her humor and insight. Her personal essence shone outward from a less than perfect face. It is easy to see the sparkling peach luck in the eyes and the smile in the photograph of Roosevelt as an older woman.

All of us had sparkling peach luck once upon a time. We were all children filled with awe and wonder about the world; just check your baby pictures. You are bound to see sparkling peach luck there somewhere. Remember what it felt like to be a playful child? If you have forgotten, it is possible to recapture that joyfulness. Watch some children and see how they play. There's a lesson there: Take life lighter. Add humor to the serious business of living. Make fun of yourself and laugh at your mistakes. Be willing to be silly. Find the child inside of you and let that child come out to play again. Be friendly. Flirt in a harmless way. Just have more fun!

If life has made you sad, you have the ability to be sympathetic and supportive of those you love. This is what is required to have supportive peach luck. Help other people, especially those you don't know. For when supportive peach luck goes beyond your immediate circle, it makes the world a kinder place by example. Be willing to listen, hug, and console. Take care of the people you love and randomly care for people you barely know, just because your heart is open. Show compassion to others the way that you would like to be treated when you need this kind of warmth. Be of service to others. Care!

Imagine what life could be like even if it is not that way now. Dream! Believe in your dreams and get others to believe in theirs. Know that the world can be made a better place if you have a plan. Don't listen to all the gloom and doom prophets and grieve for what you don't have. Instead, create possibilities in your mind and share these visions with those who need to believe too. Let the mind be free and the heart will follow. Small successes on the way to an imagined future are signs of that vision becoming true. Hold them close as evidence of what is possible. Be careful of being overwhelmed by negativity and stay away from dream killers. Making dreams come true requires persistence and faith.

So, you have suffered. Good—you have now broken down the armor that shielded your soul. This has forced you to go deep within to find out what really matters to you. You have been places in your sorrow and grief that some people have never experienced, and this has made you wise. Share this wisdom with others who don't yet know that they too can survive the fall and come out stronger. Seductive peach luck is about depth of experience in emotional pain and the lessons learned from living there. It is a mirror of resilience to those who are too afraid to go down where you have been and don't believe that they will come back.

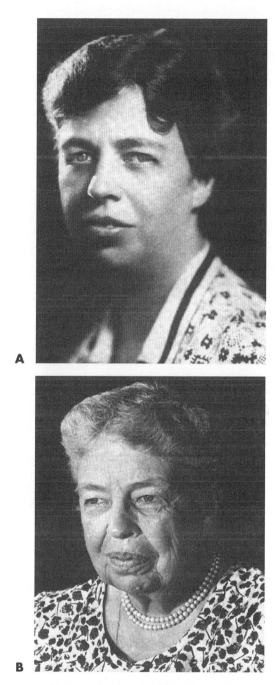

A

B

FIGURE 8-1.   This is a woman who did not have much peach luck when younger **(A)** who showed a lot of peach luck when older **(B).** In photos 51 years apart, it is evident that Eleanor Roosevelt developed sparkling, supportive, and direct peach luck. Her laugh lines and the expression of her mouth show barely contained fire; her gaze is focused, but her cheeks and lips are warm and friendly. She grew to be comfortable with herself as she grew older and showed the world many more facets of her personality.

Show them you are better for having come out the other side of the darkness that felt as though it was never going to end. Reveal how you love life all the more for knowing how precious real pleasure is and luxuriate at the end of a long journey back to yourself.

Now you know what you want. Go for it! Don't let anyone get in your way if you know that it is right for you. Those who are supposed to come along will. The rest will just get out of the way. The best use of direct peach luck is not about anger. It is about the determination to get what you want and go where you are supposed to go. It is an incredible ability to focus with the single-mindedness that leads to success and achievement.

People with direct peach luck have what the ancient Chinese called "fire and focus." A high degree of fire that is focused is one of the major signs of success. The people who possess this energy feel that they have a sense of mission. They have clear objectives that they are passionate about and disregard fear, rejection, or pain along their way to achievement. Even if there is not a lot of fire, the important aspect is the focus of whatever fire is available. This still leads to success. The single-minded pursuit of goals is admirable but can be harmful to others if the feelings of others are disregarded. The danger to those with direct peach luck is in believing that happiness comes only from success or achievement. These individuals need to remember to live and enjoy life during the journey there. This brings us back full circle in the five elements to sparkling peach luck.

Peach luck is the multifaceted expression of the soul's essence trying to express the joy and fun in life, the empathy and sympathy of the supportive person who still wants joy for others, the wistfulness and hope for dreams to come true some day, the depth of emotion and the comprehension of the mysteries of life, and the focus and determination to get what you want and the power to get it. Ultimately, though, we are capable of expressing all five types of peach luck as we get old enough to experience life and learn our lessons. Some ways of being are unsafe and not rewarded. Even though babies love to laugh, parents want to comfort their children, disillusioned adults still want to dream, deep people want to experience life's drama, driven people know what they want and how to get it, the soul's desire is to get back to the innocent self and the expression of sparkling peach luck.

Instead of becoming multidimensional and creating a spiral existence in which we get better and better as we learn more about ourselves, many people default into one form of peach luck. This is because a certain style of behavior has worked in the past. It becomes part of our signature expression of self. It can be used in negative ways and is often a technique that is used to manipulate others. To come back to your true self, discover what brings out your fire energy and use it in the way that fits you best. Eventually, learn to access all the forms of peach luck by going around the five-element wheel. This will help you manifest peach luck, but remember to do so with the best and most positive intent. Peach luck then becomes magical and beneficial. You can learn to go all the way around the peach luck cycle and end up coming back to your self—whole. This is becoming multifaceted; you adapt the expression of your fire to the circumstances. This is the chameleon that doesn't change shape, just its colors. Peach luck is like different shades of the rainbow. The rainbow is most beautiful when all the colors are present.

9 / *Facial Diagnosis*

"According to Chinese physiognomy, each area of the face corresponds to a particular organ, so a disharmony in that organ affects the complexion, texture, or moisture of the corresponding facial area."
TED J. KAPTCHUK, *THE WEB THAT HAS NO WEAVER*[1]

The oldest and first use of face reading in China was to diagnose illness from the face. The ancient healers and acupuncturists evaluated numerous small signs on the face to determine the health and current functioning of the internal organs. They first checked the *shen* by looking at the color of the skin and the light of the eyes, and then they checked each area of the face for changes in the shape, size, and markings of each feature. They correlated this information with other forms of diagnosis including looking at the tongue and checking the pulses. Only then would they treat what they saw and evaluated.

Because each area of the face is connected to the various internal organs, many health conditions can be seen in the early or preventable stages. It is then possible to help steer a person away from a disease that he or she is headed toward. The facial markings can show potential problems long before blood tests, MRIs, or CT scans can detect the problem, but the signs are subtle and must be looked at in totality and from a baseline of individual normalcy.

Diagnosis using the clues on the face is not literal, although it is based on specific information. The flesh tells a tale with subtlety and sends you from one area to another to collect all the corollary signs. The interpretation of this information requires synthesis that is based on experience. Facial diagnosis is not about looking at a face and announcing, "You have diabetes!" Instead, the face shows that there are problems with blood sugar regulation, usually involving a depression in the bridge of the nose with discoloration that signifies stagnation of the earth

---

[1]Kaptchuk TJ: *The Web That Has No Weaver,* Chicago, Congdon & Weed, 1983.

element. A practitioner would then want to look for other signs of earth excess or stagnation on the face to determine how severe this condition is or has become. At that point, it would be advisable to validate the initial diagnosis with other tests and diagnostic techniques.

Many conditions look similar to start with. Inflammation shown in the areas of the heart on the face can be a symptom of any of several different conditions from arteriosclerosis to neurological problems. It depends on where the inflammation causes harm, and that is dependent on the strength or weakness of that individual's body. No two people have the exact same disease. People can become ill from the same infection or external pathogen but can manifest the disease in very different ways, just as people react very differently to the same situation.

Facial diagnosis is a tool that instigates the exploration of the signs on the face for health purposes. It must be remembered that in ancient Chinese medicine, people were not diagnosed with diseases at all; they were diagnosed by excess and deficiency of the organs, and these various conditions were given descriptive names. The ancient healers treated symptoms, not diseases, and looked at the body and mind in totality, not as separate entities.

The ancient Chinese medical practitioners always included personality characteristics shown on the face as part of their diagnostic procedure. They believed that people with nervous temperaments or volatile emotions were very likely to have diseases that corresponded to their unique psychological makeup. The overuse of any emotion or any part of the body can take a drastic toll over time, creating illness and disease as the body breaks down. There are very few things that you can control in life, but you can have some control over your actions and reactions. Finding that middle path of living—not too much or too little expenditure of *qi*—can keep you healthy. Let's look at the signs on the face that show overuse and underuse of the emotions and the organs and what constitutes right use of the emotions and the body.

BIOLOGICAL BLUEPRINT OF THE BODY

Every major organ has a group of features that show how well that organ is functioning, either physiologically or emotionally. Heredity plays a part in determining the original strength of the organ and how well it functions. However, choices we make every day in how we feel, think, or act can also affect any organ. Over time, the reliance on certain emotions or parts of the body at the expense of others is dangerous. Underuse is just as dangerous. One of the hardest aspects of diagnosis is learning how excess and deficiency look very similar but have different underlying emotional needs involved. The other important thing to remember is to get a baseline of each person's normal state or a setpoint of each feature. This may involve looking at old photographs to determine the original genetic structure and any changes in shape that have occurred. Easiest to see are changes in the coloration of each feature. The five-element color scheme is as follows: black or gray is stagnation or stagnant water, green is toxicity or a sluggish liver that is not detoxifying, red is inflammation or an overactive heart or nervous system or trapped fire, yellow is putrefaction or things staying in the body too long, especially in the stomach, and white is frozen or a lack of energy or poor exchange of air in the lungs. The most commonly seen colors on the face are black, red, and white. Toxicity and putrefaction often are seen together as a yellow-green color (like the color of jaundice) but show up on the face less often because the liver is usually so good at detoxification.

When these colors show up in the areas correlated with each organ, they can signify either a physical or emotional problem. Distinguishing between the two can be accomplished only by questioning. For example, the area between the eyebrows is correlated to the liver. Redness in this area shows inflammation of the liver that can be caused by a pathogen or emotional irritation and anger. Either condition affects the liver. Also, if the liver is dealing with a pathogen, it can make a person more irritable or angry. Conversely, a person who is angry and irritable is much more likely to be affected by a pathogen. As you can see, the emotions and the functioning of the organs are intertwined (Tables 9-1 and 9-2). Let's look at the specific kinds of markings on the face associated with each organ.

KIDNEY SYSTEM

The ancient Chinese called the kidneys the "Minister of Power." They are the holders of the primordial *yin* energy and the first organ to develop and the last organ to fail. They are the reservoir of *jing*, the prenatal energy we came in with. Managing this *jing* is considered the most important part of longevity. The associated organs in the system are the adrenal glands, the reproductive organs, the brain and spinal cord, and the bladder. Any problems with the kidney system increase the feelings of fear, panic, and paranoia and decrease the ability to show courage, use the will, or find wisdom.

The first place to look at fundamental kidney strength is the ears. The ears are considered the best place to determine *jing*. This is the inherited constitutional strength that we live on throughout our lives. Strong *jing* is seen in firm yet flexible cartilage. Too much firmness and too little strength are both considered *jing* challenges. Major changes in the structure of the ear also indicate a weakening of the *jing*. This can be from incidents in childhood that create issues. The fear that occurs from these traumas and the energy spent attempting to avoid similar experiences happening again freezes the *jing*. This *jing* is not lost, but it is not accessible again until the person identifies, clears, and steps out of the repetitive cycle of living and gains insight and wisdom from personal experiences.

Next, look under the eyes to monitor current kidney functioning. Any noticeable depression of the skin between the cheekbone and under-eye area is a sign of dehydration. When the skin is also papery and dry, it is a further indication of a lack of water in the body. If this area is hollowed and dark, it is a sign of chronic dehydration that may have a variety of causes. It is very often associated with allergies, which are very dehydrating. However, because the lines over this area indicate lost loves, one of the primary causes of dark circles is old emotional pain from heartbreak that has not been resolved. The Chinese term for this area is

TABLE 9-1   Health Aspects*

	水	木	火	土	金
	Water	**Wood**	**Fire**	**Earth**	**Metal**
Organ	Kidney	Liver	Heart	Stomach	Lungs
Facial	Ears	Eyebrows	Eyes	Mouth	Nose
Features	Undereye	Temples	Tips and corners	Upper lip	Cheekbones
	Philtrum, Chin	Jaw		Lower cheek	Skin
Body Parts	Brain	Gallbladder	Small intestine	Pancreas	Upper back
Influenced	Spinal cord	Neck/head	Arteries	Spleen	Shoulder
	Bones	Tendons	Eyes	Muscles	Colon
	Hips	Ligaments	Hands	Midback	Nose
	Knees, ankles	Small muscles	Chest/ribs	Lips	Sinuses
	Bone marrow	Iris of eye	Complexion	Mouth	Bronchi
	Head/pubic hair	Eyebrows	Tongue	Eyelids	Skin
	Teeth	Vagina	Corners of eyes	Lymph	Mucus and
	Inner ears	Clitoris	Blood	Saliva	membranes
	Pupil of eye	Penis	Perspiration	Diaphragm	Body hair
	Ovaries/testes	Nails	Hands		
	Bladder, anus				
Disorders,	Growth	Coordination	Cardiovascular	Digestion and	Respiratory
Health	Genetic	Locomotion	diseases	absorption	disorders
Issues,	Aging	Fibromyalgia	Disturbances of	problems	Airborne
Diseases	Infertility	Migratory pain	speech and	Lymphatic	allergies
Associated	Impotence	Tension	thinking	Circulation	Shortness of
with	Miscarriage	Cramps/spasms	Insomnia	Veins	breath
Elements	Loose teeth	Irritability	Arrhythmia	Indigestion	Coughing
and	Deafness,	Nausea	Tachychardia	Flatulence	Excessive
Organs	tinnitus	Headaches	Restlessness	Poor appetite	phlegm
	Thinning hair	Irregular menses	Inflammatory	Overeating	Vulnerability
	Multiple sclerosis	Tendinitis	conditions	Anemia	to colds/flu
	Muscular	Accidents	Scatteredness	Hemorrhoids	Slow healing
	dystrophy	Liver spots	Phobias	Bruising	of skin
	Cerebral palsy	Depression	Lupus	Reflux	Emphysema
	Diseases of spinal	Substance abuse	Rheumatoid	Ulcers	Asthma
	column	Chronic fatigue	arthritis	Anorexia	Tuberculosis
	Osteoarthritis	Parkinson's	Psychosis	Bulimia	Psoriasis
		disease	Epilepsy	Crohn's disease	Pulmonary
		Repetitive strain		Cancer	diseases
		disorders (e.g.,		Diabetes	
		carpal tunnel)			

*This listing is intended to demonstrate elemental/organ connections. Some disorders and diseases, however, have multiple causes and multiple elemental involvement.

TABLE 9-2   Leading Causes of Death (1998)

		水	木	火	土	金
Disease	**Number Recorded**	**Related Issues**	**Negative Emotions**	**Healing Actions**	**Organs Involved**	
Heart disease	724,859	Abandonment Lost love Adrenalin addiction	Loneliness Lack of joy Anhedonia (lack of feeling)	Intimacy Play Living now	Heart	
Cancer* (Malignant) (Neoplasms)	541,532	Other–directedness Following rules	Overnurturing Worry Confusion	Caring for self Instinct Right action	Spleen/ stomach	
Strokes (Cerebrovascular)	158,441	Pressure Resistance	Repression Giving up	Expression/ creativity Accepting change	Kidney, liver	
Bronchitis, emphysema, asthma	112,584	Sorrow Grief	Suffering Living in the past	Positive future Finding passion	Lungs	
Accidents/ injuries	97,835	Going too fast Rashness	Rebellion Impatience	Self-awareness Slowing down	Liver, heart	
Pneumonia, influenza	91,871	Boundaries Oversocialization	Feel attacked Tribal consiousness	Redefining self Taking control	Lungs	
Diabetes	64,751	Demand for nurturing Overdependence	Bitterness Resentment	Giving Sweetness of life Self-fulfillment	Spleen/ stomach Liver	
Suicide	30,575	Disassociation Disempowerment	Escapism Futility	Life purpose	Liver, lungs	
Kidney disease (nephritis)	26,182	Will Destiny	Fear of stillness Fear of knowing	Acceptance of this life	Kidneys	
Liver disease	25,192	Absorbing toxicity Defensiveness Frustration	Anger Hostility Hate	Achieving goals Active causes Trust	Liver	

*Each form of cancer has additional issues and emotions. For example, breast and prostate cancer have gender issues.

"unshed tears." It means that there are many tears to cry and no water left to cry them. The lighter the color, the newer the pain. Pink is very recent, purple is older, and dark gray or black is very old pain. If the entire eye socket seems dark and shadowy, it is a sign of potential kidney disease. Patients who are treated with dialysis have extreme darkness under and around the eyes. This is a sign that the kidneys are not filtering waste properly and that the balance of fluids in the body is significantly off.

The most important thing to treat is the dehydration to attempt to balance the body fluids. However, drinking water alone is not the antidote. Holding in the necessary water is more important than continuing to pour it in. The current misconception is about how much water you should drink. Water is not the only answer. Many times people are drinking too much water but are not holding it in to be used by the body. To heal the kidneys, first you need rest, including doing nothing or meditating. Next most important is sleep. This is when the kidneys rest and the body heals itself. Eating foods with a high water content, such as fruits, vegetables, and soup, is also important. The minerals in these foods help bind the water in the body. The last important treatment is drinking water; here, the quality of water is important. All of the societies in which people live the longest have one striking thing in common—highly mineralized glacier water.[2] This is considered optimal drinking water because of the purity of the aerated water and the quality of the colloidal mineral content. Spring water is also considered very good, and collected rainwater is good. Water that has traveled long distances in pipes or aqueducts has lost some of its valuable *qi,* and the use of disinfectants also takes away some of the intrinsic healing properties of good water.

Bags under the eyes reveal water retention or edema in the body. This area is often white in color because of the frozen nature of the kidneys. This is a sign of fear retention or excess mineralization, which leads to the retention of water. When it is determined that the bags or puffiness under the eyes is related to fear, it usually indicates a person who is in a state of hidden panic, something I call "running away by standing still." This kind of person is usually immobilized by a secret fear and, instead of acting, does nothing to move forward except to wait and watch. It is advised that some action be attempted to move the *qi* and keep stagnation from occurring. When the body gets involved, it is a sign that the body is not processing water correctly. Water is being held, most often by a surplus of minerals left in the body. Before using diuretics, it has been found to be helpful if people with this condition drink distilled water for a short period so that the excess minerals bind to the demineralized water and are removed from the body. Because this condition can recur easily, this may need to be repeated whenever the bags reappear. A long-term consequence of overmineralization is kidney stones; when these occur, they cause severe darkness around the eye, signifying a blockage of the kidney system that has led to stagnation.

The lower eyelid is the best place to check the functioning of the adrenal glands. If the rim of the lower eyelid is red, it is a sign of aggravated adrenals. This is caused by excessive stress or sexual activity. Drooping lower lids, which causes the condition known as three-white-sided eyes, are a major sign of adrenal deficiency. People with this condition are touchy and temperamental because

---

[2]Flanagan P, Lloyd KP: Hunza water, Proceedings of the National Hydrogen Association, 10th Annual U.S. Hydrogen Meeting, *Technology Advances,* Vol 10, 1999.

their adrenals are near exhaustion. When the upper eyelids are held raised up to create the three-white-sided eyes, it is a sign of a chronically overly alert sympathetic nervous system or excessive fear and hysteria. Four-white-sided eyes are symptomatic of a hyperactive sympathetic nervous system that damages the adrenals and can lead to an early death.

The kidney system is also responsible for fertility. In fact, the ancient Chinese called the testicles the "outer kidneys." The philtrum is the area that reveals signs of fertility. This area indicates by its width and depth the potential for fertility and potency. A full and deep philtrum is a sign of strength in the reproductive organs and shows that this person is very fertile. A groove that is shallow, narrow, or marked is a sign of compromised fertility or weakness in the reproductive organs. However, this area is also the area that indicates potential creativity and spirituality. One of the strongest markings on the philtrum is a horizontal line that cuts across the groove like a bridge over a stream. This is a sign of cutting off fertility as a conscious choice or as a biological necessity caused by miscarriages or in menopause. This allows the energy that would have been used in procreation to be used instead for creation. In addition, one of the ancient Taoist beliefs was that it is much easier to become spiritual once the biological urges have been tamed and controlled, so women after menopause had an easier time becoming enlightened.

When the philtrum is discolored, it shows that the condition of the uterus and ovaries in women and the prostate and testicles in men are compromised. Redness is a sign of inflammation; for women it is usually a sign of ovulation, pregnancy, excessive bleeding, or an infection. In men it is most likely a symptom of an enlarged prostate or burning feelings with ejaculation or urination or too much sex. Darkness is a sign of stagnation. This could be caused by poor blood flow during menstruation, clotting, or the cessation of menstruation. Darkness combined with puffiness can be seen when a fibroid tumor is present. In men, darkness is often present with an inability to ejaculate, in impotence, or if there is a tumor in the testicles or prostate. White is a sign of frozenness. This is what the Chinese call a cold womb. There is a lack of blood flow and warmth to the reproductive organs, which inhibits fertility and the sex drive. In men, it occurs most often during periods of celibacy or low sperm production.

The chin is the place to look for future kidney strength. This is the area that shows the will, including the will to live. Whenever the chin shows weakening of the structure or the flesh, the will has weakened, fear has increased, or the kidneys are tired. This is most commonly seen in sagging skin around the chin or dimpling of the flesh that gives it an appearance like an orange peel. This is a classic sign of kidney deficiency in older age. Darkening in this area is an indication of increased fear, which often accompanies aging. Very often, the chin weakens after retirement because the will to work is no longer needed. A smaller chin is not necessarily a sign of a shorter life if the person with a small chin retires. A person with a strong or large chin is less likely to retire or, if forced to, will find other things to do that are treated as a career. They also have the ability to will themselves into living a long time even as their bodily functions start to deteriorate. These kinds of people have an amazing will to live and the courage to live through anything.

There are some corollary places to look for kidney deficiency. Any inherited genetic defect or developmental problem is viewed as constitutional kidney deficiency. The quality and amount of hair on the head is examined for this; lots of hair shows strong kidney energy, and thinning hair shows weakening kidney energy. The ability to hear is also an indicator. Deafness and tinnitus, or ringing in the ears, are both signs of kidney deficiency. Additional signs include low back pain and conditions of the spinal column including osteoarthritis. Kidney deficiency can also be found when there are problems with the sphincter muscles of the body, particularly the bladder, and problems with the bones and teeth, including osteoporosis and chronic knee, hip, and ankle injuries or premature aging.

To build the kidney system energy back up, learn to do nothing. Become still more often, and you will gain energy. Rest, meditate, sleep, and commune with the cosmos. Don't do so much, don't move so fast, don't feel too deeply, don't think so many thoughts, and don't live so hard. Just "be," and your kidneys will help you live a longer and wiser life.

LIVER SYSTEM

The liver in Chinese medicine is called the "General" or the "Minister of War." It is the domineering leader of the body that is responsible for war against invaders. It is the strategist that determines the best form of fighting. It also takes care of detoxification, cleanup, and rebuilding of the body when the battle is done. The liver is in charge of both growth and repair. The liver regulates the use of metabolic energy, the coordination of small muscle activity, and the functioning of the ligaments and tendons. The associated organs and the body functions of the liver system are the gallbladder, the head and neck, the sexual organs, and the eyes.

The first place to look for constitutional liver strength is the eyebrows. Thick, wiry, or coarse eyebrow hairs and long or wide eyebrows all indicate a powerful liver. All of these are signs of enhanced drive, athleticism, anger, passion, or aggression. People with big eyebrows are capable of big anger and scary aggression, and even when this anger is repressed, it has a threatening quality to it, much like a volcano that could blow at any time. However, they have more than enough strength to keep the energy down and usually prefer to let it out in myriad ways, physically or in smaller quantities. These kinds of people have tremendous physical energy and enjoy using the body. They feel betrayed by their own bodies when they break down because of overuse. Any change in the eyebrows caused from the hair falling out or thinning is indicative of a weakening liver. The strength of the liver also indicates the ability to use toxic substances, whether drugs, herbs, alcohol, or anger. Addiction can be a problem with a strong liver, and the charge gained from toxic substances or emotions can easily become a self-destructive cycle. The liver enjoys a good fight but can be overused to the point that life becomes an endless dramatic battle, and the liver wears out. Problems with depression and immobility from ensuing physical ailments are common. However, the liver is also the organ that enjoys regenerating the most and, after a rest, can come back with more energy to once again be used to do something.

When the eyebrows are naturally sparse, thin, or soft, there is much less liver *qi* to begin with. People with little eyebrows have trouble with any form of toxins, either environmental or emotional. They do not manage anger well and tend to have short fuses and minor blowups frequently. There is little power behind their words, and their anger tends not to feel very threatening. In fact, anger usually exhausts them. If the eyebrow hairs grow stronger and become coarser or appear in larger quantity, the liver *qi* is rising. This often happens after the liver cleanses or after a sustained period of assertiveness, which is good for the liver. This creates an increased ability to fight and a feeling of mild exhilaration afterward. Eyebrows can be quite easy to grow when the liver is strengthened.

The next areas to examine are the sclera, or white of the eye, for the current physical liver function and the seat of the stamp area between the eyebrows for the emotional liver function. The first thing to assess is the color. Best is a clean off-white. This is a sign of a highly functioning liver. If the sclera is blue-white, it is a sign of an underactive or frozen liver. If the eye whites are red, veined, and dry, it is a sign of liver inflammation, usually caused by overwork, physically or mentally; strained eyesight, which also overtaxes the liver; or too much anger. Eye whites that are yellow-gray-green, which looks like the color of an egg yolk next to the white, are a sign of liver toxicity. This is a combination color indicating stagnation and putrefaction along with the toxicity and is a sign of a very distressed liver. This is a common sign seen under the lower eyelid right before a person comes down with an illness like influenza or pervasively when cirrhosis of the liver has occurred from alcoholism, drug addiction, or chronic hepatitis.

Vision is also a function controlled by the liver. Blurred vision is a sign of temporary liver deficiency. This is often caused by tiredness or overuse of the eyes, but the deterioration of vision is associated with the liver energy's effect on the brain, which can create delusions because of an unwillingness to see things as they are. Such a condition is often called *denial* or a *self-induced altered state of perception*. If vision problems are indeed tied to altered states, it becomes necessary to check out the temples as well.

The temple area, as previously explained, is called the "desire for altered states." Any indentation here is a sign of this desire, whereas a fullness of flesh in this area indicates great pleasure at being human and enjoying creature comforts. The indentation, when light, belongs to a person who seeks truth and enlightenment, great creativity, and spirituality. However, if this area is dark, the person possessing this coloration and indentation of the temples shows signs of wanting to escape, whether into delusional fantasy or through drugs, alcohol, or depression. This addictive behavior is best treated by action or education, creativity, or spiritual practice.

The area between the eyebrows is a good place to get a reading on the emotional use of the liver. Markings and coloration here show how much of the various forms of anger or frustration a person has felt in the past or is currently feeling. Strong single or double lines indicate that much past anger has been felt, whether repressed or expressed, leading to a short fuse or multiple triggers, which often show up as chronic impatience and irritability. When the area is red, a person's liver is currently inflamed, and anger is present even if it is being kept controlled.

Darkness in this area is indicative of depression or exhaustion of the liver and the inability to act. A greenish color is a sign of anger that has become toxic, and white coloration is a sign of an emotionally frozen liver and the inability to express anger in any way.

The biggest problem the liver has is the creation of excessive tension that requires an appropriate outlet. Relaxation is a problem for the liver; it wants to be working constantly. Therefore the most important thing to do is to be involved in a rejuvenating activity. Many wood people rely solely on their athleticism and work out incessantly. Although this does help to relieve the tension temporarily, as does sexual release, it unfortunately creates a perpetual cycle of competition with oneself or others and ends up creating injuries of overuse. Other people use alcohol or drugs in an attempt to relax. This is actually a delusion. What appears to be relaxation outwardly is actually much work for the liver internally. Similarly, many wood-type people rely on watching sports as a relaxing pastime. In reality, their blood pressure rises, and they get emotionally involved in the game, as evidenced by their strong reactions to perceived bad calls by referees and umpires and the exultation of "their team" winning and the anger or depression caused by their team losing.

The most helpful activity for all liver conditions is to encourage outdoor exercise and activity, especially being around trees and greenery. This feeds the liver. For many people with a strong wood element, being active out in nature is a moving meditation. In addition, because of the propensity for people with strong livers to be very dramatic and do things in a big way, smaller projects involving organizing or building something are very useful. This brings the wood energy to a manageable and controllable output. Accomplishment or the satisfaction of getting things done is extremely important, and people with strong livers need to be careful about creating chaos by starting projects that are too involved or intense over prolonged periods.

To look at the functioning of the gallbladder, it is necessary to look at the length of the eyebrows. People with long eyebrows have a stronger capacity for anger, both for the short term and that sustained over time. The length of the eyebrows shows the strength of the gallbladder and the ability to digest fat and to be daring or bold in behavior. The gallbladder also aids in decision making and judgment. People with long eyebrows are more capable of feeling hate but also of turning on and turning off their anger. However, over the long term, hate is very destructive to the liver and gallbladder and is symbolized by termites living in decayed wood.

Short eyebrows are symbolic of a gallbladder deficiency. This means that individuals with these eyebrows have trouble digesting fat and prefer not to be too bold, although they can be daring on occasion. They also tend to hold onto anger in a small but constant way as resentment. This is toxic to the gallbladder over time, and the shorter the eyebrows become, the more likely a person is to be holding onto past injuries and insult, both physically and emotionally. A deficiency in the gallbladder is also evident in someone who "keeps score." Although this doesn't involve resentment, this is a simple scorekeeping system designed to keep themselves from being beholden or in debt. When resentment crystallizes, it manifests as gallstones. When resentment is taken to extremes, it is used as a weapon by which giving becomes a means of getting back, or else the desire for revenge can surface. This desire can be seen in the jaw.

The jaw is the place to look for future liver strength. This area is called "roots of the tree" for the simple reason that it shows the strength of someone's beliefs, ethics, and principles. The stronger the jaw, the stronger the bearer holds onto personal beliefs and the more willing he or she is to fight for them. This is a sign of a liver that is as strong as it now can be. When the jaw is held too tight, liver *qi* becomes excessive, and tension headaches are a common result. Temporomandibular joint syndrome or trigeminal neuralgia are also likely to occur with their associated spasms and sharp migratory pain. Long-held anger is considered a causative factor in both of these conditions. If the jaw protrudes and creates heavy jowls, the liver *qi* is very overactive. This is the trait that shows the desire for revenge and domination. When the jaw is narrow or the structure is delicate, it shows a person who is peace loving and accommodating. When the structure of the jaw weakens, as seen in sagging skin there, it is a sign of a lack of determination. If the jaw structure is involved, it shows a severe weakening of liver *qi*.

There are some corollary places to look for liver deficiency and some conditions or diseases in which this deficiency is obvious. For example, liver spots are a sign that the liver is tired. Lines and ridges or weakening of the nails can also show liver deficiency. Any condition or illness that affects mobility or coordination or locomotion, including Parkinson's disease, repetitive strain disorders, and injuries of tendons and ligaments, are all signs of overuse of the liver's energy. Other conditions that create pain, such as fibromyalgia, premenstrual syndrome, migraine headaches, muscle cramps, and spasms, also implicate compromised liver function and signify its exhaustion. Accidents are a function of liver activity as well, when rash, angry, or hurried behavior helps to create dangerous conditions.

The liver is actually a soft organ that creates a hard body. People with strong liver *qi* need to remember that their bodies and life style could use some softness too. The most common injuries, accidents, and illnesses from overactive liver *qi* come about because of rigid thinking, extreme actions, and an overactive drive. The strain and exhaustion that occur when activity is constant and the body is pushed too long ultimately result in diseases that force someone to stop, adapt, and regroup. It is wisest for people with strong livers to slow down instead of being forced to stop by their eventually rebellious bodies.

HEART SYSTEM

The heart in Chinese medicine is called the Emperor because it rules the entire body. The heart is responsible for the circulation of blood throughout the entire body and controls the expression of every emotion. This fire energy therefore touches and affects every part of the body, especially the face in the form of wrinkles. The Chinese also view the mind as part of the fire element, and thoughts are indeed fiery in nature because they involve a firing process across the synapses of the brain. The vibratory frequency of the nervous system is also involved with the fiery nature of thoughts and feelings. The associated organs and body functions of the heart system are the small intestine, the arteries, the hands, the chest and ribs, and the complexion color.

The first place to look for constitutional heart strength is the tip of the tongue. A normal tongue shows good heart *qi* when it is pale red, supple, and slightly moist. This shows normal blood flow and good vitality. As the ancient Chinese said, the tongue should have spirit. If the tongue is very pale or thin, it is indicative of blood deficiency. When the tongue is red, it shows excess heat. Purple indicates stagnation of blood, and bluing is a sign of coldness. If the tongue is swollen or very wet, it is a sign of excess dampness. If the tongue is dry and withered, this is a sign of very poor heart health. A long or narrow tongue, especially if it has a pointed tip, belongs to a very fiery person.

When the tip of the tongue is temporarily red, it is a sign of current emotional problems. Long-term emotional disharmony is seen in a pervasively red tongue. This is caused by being overly emotional or by overwork and is likely to contribute to insomnia because of the excess heat carried in the body and the mind. When there is a line through the tip, it is a sign of hereditary heart deficiency.

An alternative place on the face to look at the current functioning of the heart is on the tip of nose. This area is much easier to see and more attractive to look at and evaluate. Once again, color is the first thing to look for. If the tip of the nose is pale, there is blood deficiency or lack of blood flow in the heart or the body, which can lead to poor circulation and problems with coldness in the extremities. A nose tip that suddenly looks pinched and white could be a warning for angina pectoris. When the tip of the nose is red, it is a sign of inflammation of the emotions or some part of the body. This could just be symptomatic of excess heat held in the body or a naturally high body temperature. Small red veins on the sides of the nose indicate even more inflammatory problems in the vascular system; most likely, the arteries have been compromised by arteriosclerosis. This can also be a sign of a person with a hyperactive nervous system that contributes to difficulties maintaining a regular heartbeat (arrhythmia or tachycardia). Irregular electrical impulses of the brain, nervous system, and heart can also lead to volatile emotions, chronic anxiety, and panic attacks.

A nose tip that is purplish to grayish in color is indicative of blood stagnation or pooling of blood. This is a dangerous sign indicating poor muscle tone of the heart muscle and a possible heart attack in the near future. Another dangerous sign on the tip of the nose is an artificial puffiness of the tip that shows potential congestion in the heart or lungs. This is different from the bulbous swelling of rosacea, which also causes permanent redness of the skin. Rosacea is considered false fire. It shows as a white color underneath a splotchy redness. A line under the nose below the tip and between the nostrils indicates a hereditary heart deficiency that often just means a heart murmur was present in childhood. If a line goes through the exact tip of the nose vertically, it corresponds to mitral valve prolapse, which is considered in Western medicine to be a problem of low blood volume but was considered by the ancient Chinese to be a blood deficiency that creates a glitch in the nervous system function that controls the operation of the heart valve, not an actual heart problem. Inflammation and a red color anywhere on the face is a primary symptom of fire.

There are some corollary places to look for heart excess and deficiency and some conditions or diseases where this excess or deficiency is obvious. For example, excess fire is implicated in many diseases characterized by inflammation as a primary symptom. This includes rheumatoid arthritis, lupus, and Crohn's disease in the small intestine and other ulcerative conditions including stomach ulcers, esophageal reflux, herpes, and rashes. Heightened sensitivity to sensory stimulus is excess fire, as is an overactive imagination. Having a vivid fantasy life or active dream life is also very fiery and contributes to chronic insomnia. Excessive or inflammatory emotions that are taken to extremes can cause panic; phobias; and even psychosis, especially schizophrenia, which is characterized by paranoia, delusions of grandeur, hallucinations, and distorted speech and thinking. This mental disease starts out as fire excess and can lead to severe fire deficiency, as seen in catatonia.

Fire that has been too contained can cause an explosion. Epilepsy in traditional Chinese medicine is considered liver wind, and yet it involves a short circuit of the brain's electrical impulses. It is a like a blown fuse. Therefore I consider this condition to be excess wood that pushes into excess fire. The explosion of fire creates a backdraft, or wind, that immobilizes the body and sends it backward on the five-element cycle to wood. Interestingly, migraines are now thought to be related to misfiring of the brain as well and could be a milder condition of fire backdraft.

The pericardium is the heart protector and, when defending the heart from negative emotions, creates the feeling of tightness in the chest that is often called heart pain. This creates heart deficiency because the heart by nature is a buoyant organ and wants room to expand. The pericardium is called the "court jester" in the *Nei Jing*, or *Yellow Emperor's Classic of Medicine*, and is responsible for expressing joy. When the pericardium is healthy, the bearer has joy lines radiating upward from the outside corners of the eyes. When there are more sadness lines, going downward from the outside corners, the pericardium has usually been overactive, and the heart is being too controlled, leading to fire deficiency of the spirit.

Some syndromes and conditions of deficient fire include stammering, stuttering, and muteness. Any disconnection between the brain and the ability to communicate or receive emotions or thoughts verbally is considered a fire deficiency. Anhedonia, or the inability to feel emotions at all, is also considered fire deficiency. Autism is severe fire deficiency and metal excess; autistic individuals can tune out virtually all outside stimulation. They avoid human contact and relationships and are generally unresponsive to emotions because they have the ability to shut down due to their oversensitivity to stimulus. They are excessively metallic and need structure and order. They often have speech problems and resist change. High-functioning autism is less fire deficient and is called Asperger's syndrome. This syndrome is characterized by a lack of emotional affect and even the understanding of emotions; people with Asperger's syndrome are capable of functioning in the world in a mental way but not an emotional way. Their eyes have a kind of blankness to them, and they act in mechanical and robotic ways. The skin coloring of autistic people is usually very white and indicative of a lack of fire energy and a disconnection between the mind and the heart.

When the complexion is red, it is a sign of internal heat and lots of fire energy. These people tend to have good circulation and sweat easily, sometimes profusely. People with pale faces are fire deficient and usually have circulation problems and little perspiration. Darkness or grayness under the skin is a sign of stagnation and could be symptomatic of very poor health or a current illness.

The best place to look at current and future emotional or mental health is the eyes and the quality of light that shines through them. This light, the *shen*, is the aspect of the eyes most closely tied to the emotional heart. Diagnosing from the *shen* was and still is a highly regarded and basic form of Chinese medical diagnosis and needs to be felt as much as seen. The *Nei Jing* or *Yellow Emperor's Classic of Oriental Medicine* stated: "A doctor adept at diagnosis observes the patient's *shen*." *Shen* disturbances include problems with the emotions, the nervous system, and the brain's functioning, including difficulties in thinking and communicating. *Shen* is involved in intuition, showing joy and humor, and verbal ability. Positive *shen* is attractive and glows from the eyes. This is a sign of happiness and clarity of the mind. When the *shen* is disturbed, it is either overly bright or too dull. There are many subtle degrees of difference in the various manifestations of *shen*. According to the ancient Chinese, *shen* must be felt as well as seen. In other words, the observer has to use intuition to interpret the *shen* that is seen and to absorb the *shen* that is being displayed.

Bright eyes indicate a quick mind. There is a fast reaction time to sensory stimulation of any kind. The duller the eyes, the more slowly the brain is working, and the slower reaction time. Overly bright *shen* is considered excess fire *qi* and is seen in the most extreme cases as mania. The *shen* appears intense and hot. Mania has a wild look in which the eyes are held wide open and there is redness in the color of the skin around the eye socket and on the lower rim of the eye.

Shen that is less intense but still bright, with a vibration that feels scattered and irregular or behavior that is erratic, is a sign of hyperactivity of the brain. This is usually false fire; these people get easily overstimulated and suffer from sensory overload because they are incapable of shutting down. In even milder cases, it can be seen as flashes of overly bright light shining in the eyes and is accompanied by chattering in which the enunciation is not clear and the movements of the hands and body are erratic.

Very dull *shen* is usually a sign of mental deficiency or mental illness. The difference between the two is that the mental deficiency appears as a simple clarity in the *shen*. Mental illness, however, shows up as confused or hidden *shen*. The *shen* appears shadowed and unfocused. Pain or sadness can often be seen and felt with this type of *shen* manifestation. However, each form of mental illness has slightly different looks to the *shen*. For example, schizophrenia has a murky look (except when coupled with paranoia). In paranoid schizophrenia, the eyes get a crazed look with *shen* that sputters with an irregular vibration. Depression has a dark look, obsessive–compulsive disorder has an anxious look, and dementia has a lost look.

Shen is most attractive when life is being enjoyed. With the incidence of heart disease at its highest point ever, it is important to understand what truly heals the heart. There are many studies correlating certain emotions and activities to heart disease. In the 1970s the label "type A personality" was coined. This was a person described as being too driven, focused, intense, and angry. Later it was found that both hurrying and hostility were involved with heart disease. Eventually, Dr. Dean Ornish came up with a successful program to treat heart disease. It involved a low-fat diet, meditation, exercise, and group therapy. As he has refined his program over the years, he discovered that group therapy was one of the most healing aspects of his program and now believes that loneliness is one of the most important contributing factors in heart disease. Although the low-fat diet gets the most attention, the emotional healing that occurs during the treatment may be the most beneficial.

According to the ancient Chinese, heart failure was usually a secondary organ failure. They believed that another organ had to fail first before it affected the heart and its functioning. For example, they would look at the benefits of a low-fat diet and believe it was helping the liver system because the gallbladder digests fat properly or improperly. The liver often overacts on the heart. The special, individualized diet would also be self-nurturing and good for the spleen/stomach system. The spleen/stomach system can also overact on the heart. The ancient Chinese would view meditation as important for the kidneys, and the kidneys can and do overpower the heart energy. They considered exercise to be very important for the lungs because this helped people breathe correctly, which was the most critical component of exercising. Group therapy would be seen as good for the heart because of the exchange of emotions and verbal interaction but even more important for the spleen/stomach because of the connections and family feeling that developed. The ancient Chinese believed that the heart is best healed through the emotions.

However, the ancient Chinese believed that it was most important to control the emotions. Overindulgence in the emotions creates imbalance. They did not believe in getting too emotional about anything; in fact, they cautioned against the ups and downs of emotional expression. The sudden shifts in emotion are hard on the body and disrupt the heart's natural rhythm. They cautioned against an overactive imagination or dramatic reaction to life's circumstances. Being overly emotional or scattering the energy was considered frivolous at best and, at the very worst, dangerous. Emotional firestorms were considered a complete waste of valuable energy. They decreased the life span because they burn up so much *jing* and *qi*. The ancient Taoists recommended peacefulness, contentment, and calm behavior for longevity. They called this the "golden mean," or living in the middle of two extremes.

SPLEEN/STOMACH SYSTEM

The ancient Chinese called the spleen and corollary pancreas the "Minister of the Agriculture," and the stomach was the "warehouse" or "granary" where food was stored. These organs process, extract, assimilate, and store the nutrients that enter the body through food and drink. This system is responsible for the nourishment of the physical body, the assimilation of things from the outside, and the process of making them part of the body. The stomach is the most powerful contributor of postnatal *qi*. When the prenatal *jing* essence becomes depleted, the only way to produce more body essence is from outside forces. *Qi* is taken from the digestion of bulk food and drink. This spleen/stomach system tries to take in everything, even ideas, and make it a part of the body. Eventually, even reluctantly, the spleen/stomach system transports it for further refinement to the intestines. Therefore any problems with nourishment of the entire body, digestion of foods or ideas, or retention of nutrients or information involve the stomach. The other associated organs are the large muscles, the midback, the lymph glands, the veins, and the diaphragm. As *The Yellow Emperor's Classic of Oriental Medicine* says, "When essence is deficient, replenish it with food." Food has always been the primary medicine in the traditional Chinese system of healing.

The first place to look at to determine the fundamental spleen/pancreas and stomach strength is the mouth. This is the place where food and drink enter and are received. This means that an open mouth is receptive and a closed mouth is rejecting. Many things can be seen from the mouth regarding the health of the spleen. The spleen is in charge of muscle tone, moodiness, and metabolism. The muscle tone of the digestive organs and the body can be seen in the firmness of the mouth. Lips that are strong, full, held fairly tight, and have a firm texture symbolize strength of the spleen. This indicates good muscle tone in the body and in the digestive organs. Firm lips are an excellent sign for a singer because they show that the diaphragm muscle responsible for helping to produce sounds has strength. Singing is an earth expression of sound. The stronger the muscle tone of the lips, the bigger and more powerful the sound is that can be emitted. People with small but firm lips have reedier but clear voices. When the lips have puffiness, the voice has a grainier quality to it, and people with this trait gain weight easily throughout the body. When the lips are overly thin, the spleen is deficient. People with thin lips have trouble holding onto nutrients or material things. They have trouble gaining weight. People with flaccid lips have poor muscle tone, often accompanied by weakness in the body. They tend to overindulge in sweets and gain weight in the earthy parts of the body such as the abdominal area.

Moistness of the lips is another sign of good spleen function. Dryness signifies weakness of the spleen and a lack of fluids in the digestive tract to aid digestion. Lips that are very full, dark, or overly moist indicate spleen dampness. This is a sign of stagnation, in that the digestive organs are holding onto or retaining too much fluid and nutrients. This is a sign that can precede weight gain and accompanies obesity.

The color of the lips corresponds to blood flow and energy in the digestive organs as well as the expression of moods. Normal lips are pink or pale red in color, a sign of strength in the spleen. This shows an even temperament. People with these lips can express if they want to and hold back if they prefer. They can manage their moods and usually maintain consistency in mood. If the color of the lips is pale, it is a sign of lack of blood flow and energy in the spleen, which creates mild mood swings. When the lips are very red, there is fire trapped in the spleen.

The spleen is overactive, and the person possessing this trait is usually very moody with big mood swings. This is considered a classic sign of someone with a difficult temperament. The Chinese term for this is "having a bad spleen." In English, we often talk about "venting our spleen." Both are very appropriate expressions for the way the spleen regulates mood.

Next look at the bridge of the nose in the area directly between the eyes. This is a minor spleen/pancreas area. Worry creates the horizontal lines between the eyes and depletes the spleen and pancreas energy. The deeper the lines, the more these organs are affected. As an age marking, they also show that the body has gone through a shift or transference of energy (in the early 40s) from relying on *jing* essence, which is weakening, to instead rely more on gaining essence from food. The coloration of this area also shows blood sugar regulation. Balanced blood sugar shows as a normal, faintly pink color here. A dark bridge area shows stagnation in the digestion of sugars and carbohydrates and the possibility of diabetes. When a person is diabetic, this darkness tends to spread toward the inner corners of the eye. However, when insulin therapy is regulating the blood sugar, this discoloration will disappear. Diabetes has at its core a need for nurturing. Childhood-onset diabetes has an inherent demand for nurturing from a parent or caretaker. It requires that a caretaker monitor blood sugar, give insulin shots, and prepare proper food. In an adult, diabetes creates a demand on the self to be nurturing. This involves self-regulation and care of the disease through diet. Food was the original symbol of love and continues to be throughout life. Diabetes symbolically asks people with the disease to love themselves more.

When the area on the bridge of the nose is very pale or white, the bearer has a lack of blood sugar, which is commonly known as *hypoglycemia*. A blue color is often seen here in infants and small children and is usually a sign of lactose intolerance and an inability to break down the lactose sugars. It can also be a sign of too much sugar in the mother's diet during pregnancy or while breast-feeding.

The best place to look for current stomach functioning is above the upper lip on either side of the philtrum. This area also indicates issues about nurturing. When this area is full, clear, and pink, the stomach functioning is considered optimal, and there are few issues regarding nurturing. If this area is hollow, it indicates that stomach functioning is weak and that self-nurturing is also deficient. When this area is lined with multiple vertical lines coming from the upper lip, it is a sign of intense over-nurturing of others at the expense of oneself. The antidote to these lines and the severe deficiency in self-nourishment is pampering. When the skin in this area is overly tight, there is too much restriction on food intake. This look usually occurs while someone is on a diet. Too much control over what goes into the stomach and when food can be eaten can cause digestive disorders. The stomach is a relaxed organ and enjoys eating a variety of foods in a comfortable way. Any severe restrictions inhibit digestion because of the tension in the stomach. The most common side effects are flatulence, indigestion, or burping. The stomach's natural movement is downward; however, when it rebels, it sends energy upward, as in regurgitation.

Redness in this area is a sign of excess fire in the stomach. Eating hot and spicy foods or having an ulcer or excessive worry could cause this. If this area is white, the stomach is frozen. Drinking ice-cold beverages, eating raw foods, and partaking of frozen deserts such as ice cream most often cause this condition. The stomach is naturally the temperature of simmering soup. Anything that is not room temperature or warmer stops the assimilation process. It then takes time to reheat the stomach. Chronic coldness contributes to malabsorption and digestive distress. It is also a sign that not enough nutrients are being eaten or absorbed. Foods that build the blood are recommended. If the area is dark, stagnation of food is occurring. This is often a sign of food intolerances. When the diet becomes too predictable and repetitive, such as when the same thing is eaten day after day, the stomach can get sluggish, and the resulting inefficient digestion can lead to unnatural weight gain. The foods most likely to cause this condition are very commonly eaten foods such as wheat, dairy products, and citrus fruits. Changing the diet frequently will get the stomach energized again. When the color of the upper lip is yellowish with a hint of green, putrefaction and toxicity is evident. Some blockage in the digestive tract is forcing food to stay in the system too long. This can be a serious condition and should be treated right away.

The stomach is in charge of balancing the five tastes so that the body receives the five elements as essence extracted from the food. When the upper lip line is very refined, it is a sign of a person with a very sensitive sense of taste. Individuals with this trait balance the five tastes much more easily because they can distinguish among them so well. They dislike food that is overly seasoned. They can usually pick out the different herbs, spices, and flavors in foods. When the upper lip line is flatter and coarser, it is likely that the bearer gets stuck on one type of food as a preference at the exclusion of the others. Their ability to taste is less specific, and one flavor becomes favored because it is so easily tasted.

There are some corollary places to look for spleen/stomach excess and deficiency and some conditions or diseases in which this excess and deficiency are obvious. For example, any problems with digestion, absorption, or retention signify spleen/stomach problems. Eating disorders such as anorexia and bulimia fall under this heading. They are disorders characterized by an inability to eat enough food (anorexia) or to eat too much food and then rid the body of it (bulimia). Anorexia nervosa is shown on the face by a look of tightness in the entire mouth region. The lips are usually held together firmly, and there is a lack of color in this area. It is considered an earth deficiency of the body because of the extreme lack of food consumption, which is accompanied by rituals and habits that border on obsessiveness. Emotionally, anorexics are earthy. They tend to be pleasers, are highly conforming to society, and are dependent. These are earth behaviors. However, internally they desire self-control and start manifesting it in severe ways that start to overrule their earth personality. They are unable to give themselves the pleasure of eating. Instead, they live by rules. Bulimia is earth excess and has as its main symptoms the desire to binge on food. Afterward, vomiting or laxatives are used to rid the body of the food, so deficiency eventually does occur. Orthorexia is a newly discovered condition recently described by Dr. Steven Bratman in his book, *Health Food Junkies: Overcoming the Obsession with Healthful Eating.*[3] Dr. Bratman

---

[3]Vogt K: Doctor defines an obsession with healthy foods, calls it orthorexia nervosa: Interview with Dr. Steven Bratman, *Associated Press*, Jun 17, 2002.

believes that people who are concerned with healthy eating can become fanatic and obsessive about "good" or "healthy" food. People with orthorexia spend an inordinate amount of time thinking about food, shopping for their special food, and preparing their food in the right ways. They are obsessive about food, which makes this condition an earth excess.

Prader–Willi syndrome is a congenital earth excess characterized by children who have an insatiable desire to eat and will gorge themselves. Although they have muscle weakness that is a sign of spleen deficiency, the overwhelming desire to eat indicates an earth excess. In babies who fail to thrive, there is obviously a constitutional earth deficiency and possibly a rejection of nurturing, which is also a sign of earth deficiency.

Obesity is also an earth excess and is most often a metabolic disorder. The spleen and stomach have allowed these people to collect and hold too much earth energy. Earth people by their very nature are sedentary. Stagnation occurs easily for them. They have great fondness for sweets and starches, which are very fattening; overeating is common. Although the ancient Chinese believed that carrying some extra weight is healthy, weight becomes a problem when it inhibits mobility or creates disease.

One possible societal cause is the excessive amount of anger expressed in everyday life. Earth people become depleted from anger because, in the five-element cycle, wood vanquishes earth. If earth people are constantly bombarded with anger or other people's mood swings, they start to feel earth deficient. They then use weight as a buffer and as a way of maintaining equilibrium of their own moods; unfortunately, the pendulum often swings too far in the other direction, and they become excessively earthy. They are trying to find a balance. People with a lot of earth tend to have very consistent moods, usually fairly cheerful or at least content. Fat also buffers pain—physical or emotional. If people have been harmed psychologically in childhood because of abuse or as adults in relationships, it is likely they will turn to eating as a form of self-nurturing and put on weight to protect themselves from the pain from within or without.

Earth stagnation is also shown in the tendency for the circulation of the lymph fluid to slow or when blood coagulates too much. This is seen in such problems as varicose veins or any kind of blood clots, but particularly with clots in the leg, which are caused by thrombophlebitis. Clots are excessive earth and are also a causative factor in heart attacks and strokes. Bruising easily is a sign of earth deficiency. Bruising means there was a weakness in the walls of the veins that did not hold the blood in well when an injury occurred. Earth deficiency is also involved with prolapses of any kind, including hemorrhoids or prolapsed organs such as the uterus or other muscles such as the ones in the feet that cause fallen arches.

The area on the face corresponding to the esophagus is seen directly under the nostrils, and redness here is a sign of esophageal reflux, in which the muscles of the lower esophagus work poorly and allow reflux of the stomach contents. The redness is a sign of the inflammation and irritation that ensue. This is often related to a hiatal hernia, another condition of earth deficiency, in which part of the stomach protrudes through the diaphragm because of weak muscles in the abdominal wall.

Fatigue that includes muscle weakness and lethargy is also considered earth deficiency caused by overuse of the earth energy. It is very common when someone is a caretaker of either small children, sick people, or aging parents. This is again tied to the vertical lines on the upper lip showing too much nurturing of others. Chronic fatigue can be considered an earth deficiency as well as a wood deficiency. It usually involves overworking (taking care of business) to the point of exhaustion with very little comfort or pleasure having been allowed. Most of the recuperation involves sitting (an earth experience); eating properly, which is definitely an earth activity; and taking care of oneself or self-nurturing.

The mental component of earth is involved with the ingestion and digestion of information. When someone is unable to take in or process new information or ideas, there is an earth deficiency of the mind. This causes confusion and indecisiveness. Obsessive thinking is a form of mental earth excess. This occurs when thoughts are extremely repetitive and persistent and is considered earth stagnation. Constant worry is a milder form of earth excess.

Finally, the lower cheeks in the area known as *moneybags* is examined. This area is really representative of the reservoir of nourishment that the body is holding onto "just in case," like a savings account of *qi* to be used when needed. When this *qi* is depleted, it is very easy to get serious diseases such as cancer. Cancer is a very natural process of cell division in the body. However, when the immune system fails to recognize these cells as different, cancer begins to grow. And when cancer is present in the body, the cheek area corresponding to the lungs first gets hollow and dark, and as the cancer spreads, the lower cheeks (the moneybags area) get hollow and dark, too. This is a sign of severe earth deficiency and earth stagnation. In addition, most cancer patients also have many vertical lines in the upper lip indicating a lack of self-nurturing.

Please note that this trait alone is not a sign of cancer. Cancer is a complicated disease with many causative factors, over most of which there is little control, but studies have shown that one very distinct personality trait seems to be present in most cancer patients. It is other-directedness, or thinking of others over oneself or instead of oneself. It may also mean following the rules of society to the point of losing one's individuality. In Chinese medicine, this would definitely be considered an earth deficiency, which would lead to metal deficiency and the impairment of the immune system. Another interesting point in the treatment of cancer is the success of many of the anticancer diets being used, including the macrobiotic diet. Any change in diet that focuses on the individual and forces someone to be self-nurturing feeds the earth element and strengthens the immune system. So cancer may indeed have earth deficiency at the core. However, each specific type of cancer has other elements and personality traits involved, depending on the organ in which the cancer occurs. Cancer is not a death sentence. In fact, more and more people are surviving cancer. However, survival is not good enough. To feed the earth element, people must enjoy living.

The reserve energy shown by healthy moneybags can be saved up only if an earthy life is lived. This means paying attention to the needs of the physical body. Earth flourishes in relationship; it is the gift of companionship, comfort, and help given to others and received back in turn. Earth values pleasure, as in eating and really tasting all kinds of foods. Sit more, slow down, and nurture yourself.

LUNG SYSTEM

The lungs in Chinese medicine are named "The Prime Minister" or the "Advisor" to the Emperor (the heart) and run the day-to-day operations of the body based on respiration; they establish order in the body. The lungs have also been called the "Minister of Security" because they monitor the territorial boundaries, or the skin, which is considered the first line of defense for the body. The lung system tries to shield the body from invasion by the six pernicious influences: wind, heat, dryness, dampness, summer heat, and cold. Invasion by these influences causes disharmony and disease. The skin attempts to resist these influences and tries to protect the inner treasures by scaling off the major entrance to the body, the pores. The skin constantly monitors moisture and temperature and opens or closes the pores accordingly. The skin is often called the "third lung" because of this mini-form of breathing. Pores that are too open show vulnerability in the lung system, and pores that are too tight show an overactive defense system. When the skin is too dry, the lungs are also too dry. When the skin is pale, the lungs are blood deficient, and when the skin is red, there is inflammation and excess fire in the lungs or lung system. Blueness shows a lack of oxygen; a gray color is indicative of stagnation. Skin infections are a sign of poor boundaries. These include fungal overgrowth and impetigo. When the skin overgrows after an injury, it is a sign of excess metal and is called a *keloid*. When the skin heals slowly, it is a sign of deficient metal energy and lowered immune function.

Breathing is the most essential aspect of living. You can go without food for several weeks and without water for several days, but if you stop breathing, you only have minutes before you die. Breathing is the essential element to living. It also controls the autonomous nervous system. Controlling the breath to gain spiritual mastery has been a goal of many spiritual teachings. Breathing was considered the bridge between the mind and the body. The ancient Taoist form of breathing exercises is *qi gong*. The lungs are considered the alchemist of the body by turning breath into *qi* after combining it with the *qi* essence from food sent from the spleen/stomach system. Breathing in is called *inspiration* and expands and inflates life; breathing out is called *expiration,* which shrinks and minimizes life. The lungs are therefore involved with living and dying, even moment to moment.

Involuntary cessation of breath during sleep is called *sleep apnea.* This is a sign of lung deficiency and a glitch in the autonomic nervous system. The lung system energy is not flowing smoothly. Shallow breathing, including hyperventilation, is also considered lung deficiency. The ancient Chinese believed that the best breathing occurred by inhaling through the nose deeply and exhaling through the mouth even more deeply. This was the proper way to receive energy while inhaling and to cleanse the body while exhaling. In contrast, a yawn is just for energizing, and a sigh is just for release. Deliberate breathing to both energize and cleanse is said to balance the connection between the mind and the body.

The first place to look for constitutional lung strength is the nose. The ancient Chinese called the nose the "Gate of Breath." The size of the nose in the overview of the face is proportional to the size of the lungs within the body cavity. Bigger noses are considered to have more constitutional lung strength, whereas small noses have smaller lung capacity. How the nose functions for breathing is more important. Because the nose is the first filter for air and temperature, respiratory allergies are considered a sign of a very active immune response to seemingly innocuous and microscopic substances. This is actually a sign of very strong lung *qi,* especially when the onset of allergies occurs in childhood. As irritating as allergies can be, people with severe allergies are unlikely to get cancer, because their bodies are so good at eliminating unwanted cells and pathogens. They have an almost overactive shield to external pathogens and are very sensitive to things other people's bodies disregard. When the allergies occur later in life, or systemically in response to environmental toxins, it is a sign of lung deficiency caused by the breakdown of the shield and the early warning system.

A nose that is constantly clogged and chronically swollen sinuses are a sign of lung stagnation. Mucus production is governed by the lungs and is designed to remove and eliminate unwanted particulate matter from the respiratory system. It is intended to flow freely. This is a sign of healthy lungs. When the transmission of this fluid is blocked, the mucus congeals, and either sneezing or congestion occurs. Sneezing is a way of expelling an irritant or a mucus plug. This can restore equilibrium to the respiratory system and is initially a sign of lung strength. When sneezing becomes repetitive, it can lead to lung deficiency because so such much air is lost in each convulsive explosion. Coughing is the other way of releasing mucus.

Stagnation occurs because the lungs are unable to release mucus. This is exacerbated by dampness. This condition may be caused by the cold or a flu virus and is a sign that the defenses have been invaded. When the stagnation becomes severe, it can lead to lung diseases of stagnation, including sinusitis and bronchitis, and can ultimately lead to pneumonia or pleurisy. Chronic bronchitis is a condition of lung deficiency that often leads to or accompanies emphysema, in which the lungs are damaged beyond repair. Symptoms include shortness of breath and a chronic cough that is often accompanied by wheezing. Emphysema is seen as very pale skin with a faint blueness as a result of the lack of oxygen/carbon dioxide exchange in the damaged alveoli. The skin gets grayer and darker as the disease progresses. If the cheeks get puffy looking, it is a sign of pulmonary edema or fluid in the lungs and stagnation. Usually, however, the cheeks on either side of the mouth get extremely hollow and lined, showing the severe deficiency of the lungs, and the chest puffs out. Although air pollution and cigarette smoking have been strongly implicated as causes of emphysema, the emotional underlay of this disease indicates severe grief that is unresolved and relatively unprocessed. In my experience, people suffering from emphysema treat the loss of loved ones in the past as if their passing just happened. The grief is kept raw and current. This perpetual state of grief inhibits lung function, lowers immune function, and prevents the lungs from processing environmental toxins.

Another condition that causes shortness of breath is asthma. Extrinsic asthma is caused by allergies; intrinsic asthma is most likely based on stress and anxiety.

In Chinese medicine, asthma is considered a boundary problem. Extrinsic asthma starts out as excess lung *qi* because of the overresponsiveness of the lungs to foreign invaders. The actual asthma attack ends up causing lung deficiency, especially when attacks occur often and breathing is constantly restricted. One of the underlying factors in asthma may be claustrophobia, especially for intrinsic asthma. The reaction of people who have strong needs for space emotionally or physically can create shallow breathing that accompanies a feeling of panic. This can lead to restriction and narrowing of the bronchioles. The stronger the reaction, the more inflammatory the lungs can get. Many fatal cases of asthma occur in people who live in the inner city in very crowded conditions.

Overcrowding and claustrophobia may also lead to tuberculosis, which is also more common in deprived inner city environments and in damp climates. This is a disease of lung stagnation, as is evidenced by the overall gray color of the facial skin. Interestingly, in the 1800s and early 1900s, the best treatment was to send patients to sanitariums where the environment was extremely clean (metallic), the grounds were spacious, patients had their own private rooms, and the air was clean. The Old West was originally populated with characters seeking wide open spaces and clean air to deal with their "consumption."

The color of the mucus is the best way to tell how severe a respiratory illness is. Clear and thin mucus is a sign of lung strength. When the mucus becomes cloudy white and thick, the lungs are having trouble clearing toxins. Mucus that is yellow-green is a sign of toxicity and putrefaction. In addition, the redness of the nose and throat during a respiratory illness signify inflammation. When blood is in the sputum, the inflammation has become very serious.

Another sign of strong lung *qi* is a very sensitive sense of smell. This is seen as nostrils that look carved out or arch upward on the alae. There is a refinement to the sense of smell that allows these people to instantly interpret what they smell, identify it, and react to it. When someone loses the sense of smell, it is a sign of severe deficiency of the lung system.

A corollary tightness of the shoulders and upper back can be seen on the upper part of the nose at the place the bone ends and the cartilage begins. When the muscles are strained in this area, the skin on the nose corresponds and appears tight over the bone. This is a sign of tension in the lungs.

The large intestines is the next area to consider and is what the ancient Chinese called the "Minister of Transportation." It is more commonly called the colon. This is shown on the face in the lines that radiate down from the nose and end on either side of the mouth. These lines show whether the colon is functioning properly both physically and emotionally. When this area has a good color, the colon is in good function. The colon is the organ that determines what we want to keep in our bodies and lives and what we are going to get rid of from our bodies and lives. It decides what belongs to us and what does not. It eliminates the old to bring in the new; otherwise life stands still. A person who is unable to eliminate cannot move on.

The colon is even responsible for letting go of any unnecessary thoughts, feelings, or attachments and is easily influenced by anxiety. It is a controlling organ in that it has strict rules and regulations; it is the knife of the body. When someone is indecisive and wishy-washy, the colon can create spastic conditions such as a spastic colon. The colon is also very susceptible to blockage. Constipation is one such blockage and is considered an inability to let go. It shows up in the *fa-ling* lines as darkness. Diarrhea is caused by attempting to let things go too quickly without evaluation. The *fa-ling* area will probably be very light or pale in color. Certain conditions such as colitis, ulcerative colitis, and irritable bowel syndrome are tied to inflammation of the colon. This shows up on the *fa-ling* lines as redness. The colon also controls the release of emotional baggage. Trying to take too much baggage from the past can mark this area with stagnation and darkness and hamper movement toward the future. Lacking purpose inhibits the *fa-ling* lines from even forming at all.

The cheek area is called the "breath of life." This can be evaluated each day to determine whether a person is living in the present. A fullness and pinkness in the cheek area indicates the individual is breathing adequately for the body's needs. If this area is faintly lined or hollow, the breathing is either too shallow or too fast. If this area is faintly dark, the breathing is not bringing in quite enough oxygen and the lungs are not detoxifying fully on the out-breath. If this area is very hollow or very dark, the immune functioning has been compromised. This look usually accompanies serious disease such as cancer or emphysema, as previously discussed. It also accompanies AIDS. However, this is a disease that starts off with darkness in the breath of life area that eventually clears, maintaining the hollowness as the darkness disappears, and the facial coloring becomes very light and even radiant, perhaps indicating a spiritual transformation involving self-acceptance. AIDS is also a very metallic disease, involving the skin and the lungs in most cases.

The deeper one breathes, the more beautiful the color of the skin is, and the healthier the skin looks. The moment between breaths deserves special attention because it is the moment when time stands still, when anything is possible. This is a spiritual moment that the Taoists spent much time cultivating to expand their awareness. They called it "solidifying the breath and letting it grow." It was a practice that they used to achieve longevity.

The lungs are about the future. If you open your lungs, you are opening yourself to the future. If you close off your lungs, you only have the past. Grief and sadness about the past hold you back. You can only attain your goals when you release emotions that no longer serve you with every exhale and accept your new self with every new breath. This is alchemy, transforming yourself beyond the body to becoming a spiritual being.

Conclusion: The Wisdom of the Face

"When metal and wood, sense and essence, join together, this is the complete Original Face without defect."
CHANG PO-TUAN, *THE INNER TEACHINGS OF TAOISM*[1]

Your face shows who you are, how you have lived and felt, and who you can become. That's a lot of information packed into a very small area. The face also changes as we change and becomes who we become. The face to me is a hologram, not just of the body and its internal structure and function but really is a holographic interpretation of your soul. The *Random House Dictionary* defines a hologram as: "the three dimensional image of an object produced by recording ... the patterns of interference formed by a split ... beam and then illuminating the pattern with coherent light." The soul is the beam. The interference is our genetic structure, the issues and patterns of our personal conditioning, our personality, and our psychology. Illuminating the pattern with coherent light means that it is necessary to look beyond how we appear to be and get to the soul level of being to see who we really are. When the pattern clears, what is left to see? We see our original face.

Our original face can shine through our human face, illuminating us through the pores of our skin and through the light of the eyes. The light has always been there, sometimes seen for moments, even years. The layers of remembered experience and the issues and patterns that develop cast shadows over our internal sun. Our spirits can wither, and our faces age and sag in response. But when the light can be found, the spirit can be rejuvenated, and so can the face and body.

The cream you put on your face or the special foods you eat are not what are truly important. They do help in the rejuvenation process. Care for your body and your face because they serve you so well (Table C-1). However, what really matters is that we begin to free ourselves from the cultural conditioning about aging and

---

[1]Chang Po-Tuan: *The Inner Teachings of Taoism* (trans. Thomas Cleary), Boston, Shambhala, 1986.

207

TABLE C-1   Balancing and Healing the Body and Spirit

	Water	Wood	Fire	Earth	Metal
ORGAN	Kidney	Liver	Heart	Stomach	Lungs
PRIMARY ACTION	Be	Do	Live, play	Connect, nurture	Control, aspire
PHYSICAL HEALING ACTIONS	Hydration Good water Make soup Sleep Rest Meditate Eat salty foods Bathe, swim Find spirituality Cultivate mystical experiences	Energize life with action: exercise Become flexible Take up a cause Get something done Use herbs Eat sour foods Spend time around trees Grow things Hike, walk, work	Enjoy life Have fun Open heart to new experiences and intimacy Travel Choose happiness Try new hot and bitter foods Rediscover childlike wonder Communicate Smile, laugh, love	Be involved Nurture self Give freely Indulge in sensual pleasures of life: Garden, Make bread Keep good company Eat sweet foods Relax Hug	Stay in present Use discipline Create order Be surrounded with elegance, beauty, refinement, and manners Live by ideals Be grateful Eat pungent foods Breathe on purpose
HARMFUL EMOTIONS	Fear Willfulness	Anger Hate	Sadness Abandonment Excess excitement	Worry Confusion	Grief Lack
EMOTIONAL REACTION	Freezing/flight Stubbornness Lack of flow	Depression Responsibility Overdoing or not doing	Anxiety Nervousness Seriousness Scattered	Indecision Over nurturing under nurturing Smothering Material neediness	Perfectionism Lack of self-esteem Grandiosity Claustrophobia
TRANSCENDENT HEALING EMOTIONS	Wisdom Allowing	Human kindness Compassion	Happiness Unconditional love	Instinct Right action	Gratitude Mindfulness

beauty. Souls are beautiful, not turned-up noses and full lips—those are just attractive. Souls are timeless, and bodies are not. If we reinterpret beauty to be about how much our souls show, our age will matter as little as our shoe size does. The most beautiful people I have ever known have been people willing to show their souls to the world. Some were very young, and some were very old, but the one thing they had in common was their willingness to be real. How do you show your soul?

The path to enlightenment is an individual one. As the saying goes, "there are many paths to God." You need to find yours. It is a long and interesting journey that started long ago. It is the story of your life that has led you here. Your story has marked your face, a sign that you must revisit what you have already lived. Your patterns and issues have been using up your *jing* and aging your face and body, but these are the experiences that show you your shadows. Shine the light of truth into the darkest parts of your psyche and accept who you are and what you have done. You are human, and being human is very messy. Clean up the residue; remove the pain and the guilt and the shame.

The shadows will stop blocking the light of your soul. Your lines will begin to fall away and lessen in severity. You are freeing yourself from your patterns, and you are ready to find your Golden Path.

The Golden Path is my interpretation of the Taoist way to enlightenment. It is about discovering what you are here to do so that you can contribute something while you are here. It is a way of achieving longevity and even immortality. This is individual work that must done within. There are many practices and techniques for refining your essence. The one I give to you is called the *Transcendent Emotions*.

THE TRANSCENDENT EMOTIONS

The Transcendent Emotions are easy to understand and simple to express. They are easy to feel, but to live by them is much harder. It involves moving away from the human emotions that have helped and harmed us. They are used as protective weapons and shields that keep us warring. The transcendent emotions are spiritual emotions that regenerate us and bring us together. These emotions are one way out of the *yin/yang* matrix and into wholeness. They help clear the way for the soul to show on the face and emanate as true beauty. They are the transformations of:

- Fear to Wisdom—a look of serenity
- Anger to Human Kindness/Compassion—a look of softness
- Joy/Excitement to Love—the glow of warmth
- Worry to Right Action—the look of clarity
- Grief to Gratitude—the look of rapture

Wisdom can be gained from many places. It emerges from others when needed or can be discovered in the book that falls on your foot. It can be found in many great spiritual and religious teachings, in clichés, and in the simple words of children. I call wisdom the "Cosmic Water" that puts out the spontaneous combustion fear causes in the body. It calms and soothes and can be felt as truth.

Human kindness and compassion don't allow you to stay angry. If perpetrators of violence could feel their victim's pain, they would cease their actions. Human kindness is humanitarianism. It is about doing for others without need of reward and being of service because you care about making the world better. It transforms a personal cause into a universal action of goodness that ripples beyond the act through the power of positive intent.

Joy or excitement is really about seeking sensation. It is the act of running away from boredom and doing anything or everything to keep from feeling the letdown after the thrill. What gets people off the roller coaster ride is love (especially self-love), not romantic infatuation or need. It must be unconditional love.

Worry never accomplishes anything except to give you more worry. It is a revolving, circular energy that accomplishes little. It creates indecisiveness and inaction. The way out is through instinct. This allows for right action and shows you how to know what is right for you. You will become the expert about you. Your mind will clear.

Gratitude is the last of the transcendent emotions. There is so much grief in the world. It is a part of the unchanging human dilemma to lose the people or things that they love. It is a natural human desire to attach to others and possessions. But we truly own nothing and take nothing with us when we go. What's left is the beauty of the experiences, the trace memories of the richness of being alive. It is much better to appreciate what you've been given while you are still here. Gratitude is the most amazing emotion. It resets the autonomic nervous system with the inspiration of the first breath and helps let go of so much of our suffering with the expiration of the outbreath. Gratitude brings down the light of the divine so that it can shine through your face. It helps you live in that moment between breaths when anything is possible and you can become who you are meant to be. This is the beauty of you.

I leave you to return to my quest, to unlock the mysteries of my trinity—Universal Truth, Unconditional Love, and Intrinsic Beauty. I strive to live up to the meaning of my Chinese name, Independent Lotus Blossom (Color Plate 19). I wish you well on your path of self-discovery.

Index

Note: Numerals followed by f refer to figures. Numerals followed by t refer to tables.